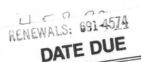

Abnormal Ageing

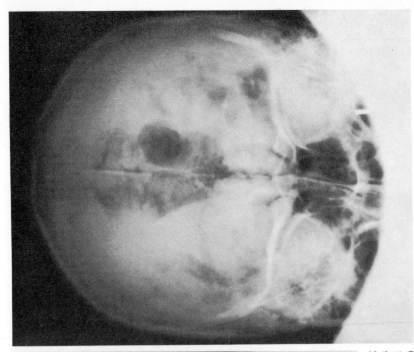

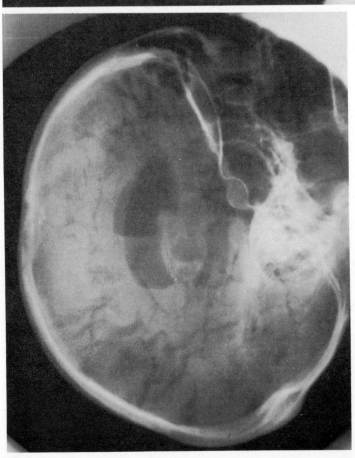

Frontispiece. Air encephalogram (with both lateral and antero-posterior views) showing cerebral atrophy. The ventricles are enlarged to an abnormal degree and there is gross 'pooling' of air in the atrophied cortical sulci over the convexities of the cerebral hemispheres. (Kindly supplied by Dr E. H. Burrows, Wessex Neurological Centre.)

Abnormal Ageing

The Psychology of Senile and Presenile Dementia

EDGAR MILLER

University of Southampton

JOHN WILEY & SONS

London · New York · Sydney · Toronto

Copyright © 1977, by John Wiley & Sons, Ltd.

Library of Congress Cataloging in Publication Data:

Miller, Edgar.
  Abnormal ageing.

  Includes indexes.
  1. Senile psychosis. 2. Presenile dementia.
I. Title. [DNLM: 1. Ageing. 2. Dementia,
Presenile. 3. Psychoses, Senile. WT150 M647a]
RC524.M54   616.8′983   76–28175

ISBN 0 471 99439 1

Photosetting by Thomson Press (India) Limited, New Delhi,
and printed by offset lithography by Unwin Brothers Limited,
The Gresham Press, Old Woking, Surrey

To
Sally, Jo, James and Andrew

Contents

Preface

The nature and extent of progress in present day psychology is open to dispute. What is in no doubt is the fact that there is rapid expansion in writing about psychology. As the author of yet another book I feel particularly obliged to justify my addition to the deluge of printed paper. Ageing is rightly a topic of current concern not only because it has been somewhat neglected in the past, but because the increasing proportion of the population who are elderly presents numerous problems for our society. Amongst the older members of the population are some whose loss of functional capacity is much greater than could be accounted for in terms of the normal ageing process. These individuals who suffer abnormal psychological changes with ageing are commonly described as having dementia and they present problems that are particularly difficult to handle.

The basic aim of this book is to present the psychological aspects of dementia as far as these are known. Although there is a diffuse literature on this topic it has never been brought together or evaluated as a whole. I hope that this will be seen as the major achievement of this book. The issues surrounding dementia are multifaceted and extend well beyond the boundaries of psychology. For this reason I have attempted, in so far as I am able, to relate the psychological aspects of dementia to the approaches of other disciplines especially those associated with medicine. Similarly the problems of abnormal ageing cannot be fully understood without an appreciation of the processes of normal ageing. As will be seen, it is not yet possible to build strong bridges between the study of dementia and that of normal ageing but I have felt it necessary, for the benefit of those readers not familiar with the psychology of normal ageing, to devote a chapter to that topic. This chapter is intended to give a general orientation to work on normal ageing and should in no way be seen as a definitive summary of the psychology of normal ageing.

As a clinical psychologist I am especially aware of the need to develop practical ways of coping with the problem of dementia. I have therefore endeavoured to deal with the practical aspects in some detail in the closing chapters. In terms of their relative predominance in the literature in general I have also tried to stress the very difficult and immediately practical problem of management at the expense of the less critical question of assessment.

My interest in dementia first began when I was a member of the staff of the Department of Psychology, University of Hull, and linked to the Combined Neurological Service, Hull Royal Infirmary. It was first inspired by Maria Ron, now at the Institute of Psychiatry in London, and John Pearce, Consultant Neurologist. Whatever merit this book may have owes much to them and to other colleagues both in Hull and in the Medical Faculty at Southampton University where I am presently employed. A debt of gratitude is also owed to the Psychology Department of Queen's University, Kingston, Ontario, who have provided me with a very congenial base for the current academic year and the opportunity to tackle the final draft of this book whilst free of my normal clinical and academic pressures. Finally I would like to record my appreciation of the efficient secretarial help offered by Joan King in Southampton and Agnes Ganchev at Queen's.

Psychology Department,   EDGAR MILLER
Queen's University,
Kingston, Ontario

April 1976.

Part One
Introduction

1
Ageing and Dementia

It is well established that in Britain, as in other Western industrialized communities, the elderly form an increasing proportion of the population. Figures given by the Office of Health Economics in London show that at the turn of the last century about 5% of the population of England and Wales were over 65 years of age. At the time of writing the proportion in this age group is around 13% and still rising. So far the dominant factor in this trend has been the lowered fertility rate in the early part of this century, although the increased life expectancy brought about by medical advances will play an increasing part in its maintenance.

It is almost tautologous to argue that an increase in the proportion of the elderly means an increase in the problems associated with old age. The demand placed upon the health services by the failing health of the elderly individual is often commented upon but there are many other less publicized causes for concern. The social role of the elderly is also undergoing change and has yet to be satisfactorily resolved. This is particularly so in an age which places an increasing emphasis on youth and when increased mobility has weakened family ties. There is also the economic strain placed upon the community in general in having to support a higher number of relatively unproductive adults.

One particular problem associated with ageing is illustrated by the word 'senile'. This adjective can be used in two different ways. Its general meaning can be defined as 'pertaining to ageing' but it has a second, more specific use to refer to the marked mental deterioration found in some elderly persons. The different uses of this word illustrate how closely we associate the mental changes found in even a normal, healthy old age with the gross and abnormal manifestations occurring in the older person with dementia.

This book is concerned with the abnormal manifestation of ageing known as 'dementia'. It is particularly concerned with the psychological aspects of dementia. These are of some importance since, despite its physical cause, the primary connotations of the term 'dementia' are psychological and the use of the term implies, above all else, a general deterioration in intellectual functioning. Despite this, and the frequency with which patients with dementia are encountered in clinical practice, there has been little sustained enthusiasm for the study of dementia by clinical psychologists. This is not to say that there has not been any work on the subject but rather that the work that has appeared has been spasmodic and uncoordinated. The aim of this book is to try to redress the balance by presenting a detailed analysis of the psychology of dementia.

Before proceeding further in this task it is necessary to attempt to answer a number of preliminary questions. These relate to such things as the meaning of dementia, how common it is, and the way in which it is diagnosed. Not until these issues are decided can we meaningfully try to establish the behavioural disturbances associated with dementia.

THE CONCEPT OF DEMENTIA

It is unfortunate that the term 'dementia' can have two meanings. It can be used in a purely descriptive sense to indicate that certain changes have occurred in a patient. For example, a patient with a localized turmour in the brain may be functioning at an intellectual level which is well below that associated with a person having his educational and social history. He may also be apathetic and take little interest in what is going on around him. Such a patient may well be described as 'demented'. In this descriptive sense the label of 'dementia' can be applied to such a wide range of neurological and psychiatric conditions that it would be inappropriate to look for an underlying unitary pattern of psychological disturbance.

The second meaning of the term 'dementia' is in a diagnostic or classificatory sense in which it is used to refer to a specific disease or group of diseases. The conditions considered to fall into the category of the dementias are commonly divided into two groups according to the age of onset. Those occurring after some arbitrary age level, often taken as 65 years, are designated senile dementias, whilst those manifest before this age level constitute the presenile dementias. The main types of dementia occurring in the senile and presenile age ranges are shown in Table 1.

Certain of the conditions listed in Table 1 can usually be set aside from the rest. Within the presenile range Huntington's chorea, Jacob Creutzfeldt's disease, normal pressure hydrocephalus and neurosyphilis are all rare forms of dementia. They can be distinguished from one another and from the rest of the dementias on the basis of special investigations, family history and characteristic motor signs.

In the past it has often been the practice, especially among psychiatrists,

TABLE 1
The main diseases associated with dementia

Presenile group	Senile group
Alzheimer's disease	Senile dementia
Pick's disease	Arteriosclerotic dementia
Huntington's chorea	
Jacob Creutzfeldt's disease	
Normal pressure hydrocephalus	
Neurosyphilis	

to assume that a very large proportion of all dementias which were not readily diagnosed as belonging to one of these rare categories were due to cerebral arteriosclerosis. Whilst it is undoubtedly true that repeated small infarcts or haemorrhages within the brain can cause dementia, recent pathological investigations (Tomlinson *et al.*, 1970) have indicated that arterioscelerosis is a major aetiological factor in only a small proportion of cases. The diagnosis of arteriosclerotic dementia is only justified where there is evidence of multiple strokes (Pearce and Miller, 1973) producing sudden exacerbations in the condition as opposed to the relatively smooth and steady decline found in most cases of dementia.

There now remains the large proportion of patients with dementia who fall, by exclusion, into the categories of Alzheimer's or Pick's disease within the presenile age range or into that of senile dementia. Distinctions can be drawn between these three conditions in theory, usually on pathological grounds, but satisfactory discrimination is impossible in practice (Pearce and Miller, 1973). In the clinical situation Alzheimer's disease can only be distinguished from senile dementia on the very dubious grounds of an arbitrarily-fixed age level. Pick's disease, even if it exists as a distinct entity, is very rare and similarly very difficult to separate from Alzheimer's disease in life. These three conditions all have one important and overriding feature in common: they are all associated with cerebral atrophy for which there is no established cause. As Pearce and Miller (1973) have suggested they might be more accurately described 'primary cerebral atrophy'.

It is with this type of dementia that the present book is concerned. Where the term 'dementia' is used in future in this book it will refer to primary cerebral atrophy. Dementia in this slightly narrower use of the term as a diagnostic label, will include by far the largest proportion of demented patients. It is being assumed that patients with primary cerebral atrophy form a homogeneous group. In the writer's opinion there is no convincing demonstration that this assumption is invalid. Even if it is ultimately shown to be invalid, the pathological changes that all cases of primary cerebral atrophy have in common would still make them a relatively homogeneous group. Any differences within the category of dementia defined in this way would probably be small as compared to the differences between patients with dementia and either normal subjects or other diagnostic groups. It is therefore reasonable to look for psychological characteristics attributable to this type of patient.

CLINICAL DESCRIPTION OF DEMENTIA

At a descriptive level the patient with dementia has a number of functional disturbances. Early on in the illness the most prominent of these is usually an impairment in memory. This shows as a failure to register events. Recall of the patient's past life is relatively well preserved but recent occurrences are forgotten. Often this is first noticed in the course of daily activity. The clerk forgets to document transactions in the appropriate way and the housewife returns from her shopping having failed to purchase the necessary items that she had intended to obtain.

There is always a general deterioration in intellectual functioning. The patient's ability to grasp issues becomes reduced and his thinking gradually more concrete and impoverished. Routine activities may be carried out reasonably well at first but anything that requires an understanding of new, or even slightly revised, principles is extremely difficult. Although it is an essential feature of dementia, intellectual deterioration may not be the most obvious feature in the earliest stages of the illness.

Emotional changes, especially depression, are common in the early stages of a dementing illness and may even be the presenting symptom. The patient may be withdrawn, retarded in speech and movement, gloomy, neglectful of himself, and have feelings of inadequacy. This picture can often be confused with an endogenous depression. On the other hand, a state of fatuous euphoria is occasionally seen. The patient remains oblivious of the changes that are taking place and is cheerfully confident of his ability. He is at a loss to understand why his relatives and friends are so worried about him and regards their endeavours to get him to take medical advice with an amused tolerance. This state is not like hypomania in that some essential hypomanic features such as over-activity and pressure of talk are not found. As the illness progresses the mood changes to one of apathy regardless of its initial state.

Dementia also produces changes in personality. These can be quite varied and are difficult to summarize succinctly. Sometimes an exaggeration of premorbid traits occurs. The person with slight obsessional tendencies becomes over-fussy and displays rigidity and frankly obsessional signs. Sometimes the reverse process may occur in which the premorbid personality becomes grossly changed or its prominent features even reversed. Here the quiet, introverted individual may become disinhibited, loud mouthed, boastful and aggressive. The loosening of inhibitions is particularly likely to be a source of worry to relatives because the patient may indulge in socially unacceptable behaviour without any appreciation of the distress it causes others. Again these are the changes that may be evident at the time when dementia is first suspected. Eventually the marked features of the personality will fade and it will become flat and colourless.

In addition to these specifically psychological manifestations there is likely to be a whole range of neurological or neuropsychological features. Disturbances akin to aphasia are quite common as the illness develops but may also be present in the early stages. The first changes in language are usually a restricted vocabulary and range of expression but more classical features of dysphasia, such as nominal dysphasia, may be elicited later. Demented patients also develop agnosias and apraxias. Constructional apraxia is usually particularly easy to demonstrate. Recently it has also been shown that extrapyramidal signs can be found in a majority of early cases of dementia (Pearce and Miller, 1973).

Dementia is a progressive condition. Typically, it first shows itself as a difficulty in memory or in affective changes. Sometimes an initial depression is so marked that the patient will be regarded, initially, as having this alone. Gradually the deterioration in cognitive functioning becomes more and more marked and the patient becomes apathetic and disinterested in his environment. In the final stages there is a complete breakdown in intellect and personality and the patient requires extensive care to cope with such things as double incontinence.

PATHOLOGY OF DEMENTIA

A detailed exposition on the pathology of dementia would be out of place in this volume. A brief outline is all that is called for and indeed all that the author is capable of giving. A much more extensive presentation can be found in Pearce and Miller (1973). In general, the pathological changes that occur in dementia are not unique to this condition but can be found in the normal ageing brain. The brain of the demented patient is thus distinguished from that of the normal older person by the extent of the change that has taken place rather than by its nature.

The most obvious pathological change in dementia is the atrophy of the brain. The total brain weight is reduced, the gyri are shrunken with consequent widening of the sulci, and the ventricles are enlarged. Microscopically the major features are the occurrence of senile plaques, neurofibrillary tangles and granuovacuolar changes. The most extensively studied of these are the senile plaques. These are commonly found with advancing age in the normal brain but are especially prevalent in the dementing brain. They are found most prominently in the frontal, temporal and hippocampal cortex. The frequency of these plaques, which may well result from neuronal degeneration, has been found to correlate with intellectual deterioration (Corsellis, 1962; Roth et al., 1967).

The fact that the major pathological changes associated with dementia can be found in the normal ageing brain lends support to the commonly expressed notion that what we see in dementia is the effect of an accelerated ageing of the nervous system. This theory will be discussed in greater detail in a later chapter but it should be noted here that the pathological similarities between dementia and normal ageing do not prove that the processes are identical, although they are consistent with the theory. There are also a few neuropathologists (e.g., Dayan, 1971) who are convinced that the similarity stops short of identity. In any case it is possible that the same pathological changes could be produced by different causal agents. Furthermore the pattern of these different changes relative to one another may be different, thus producing different behavioural consequences.

EPIDEMIOLOGY

As was the case in presenting the pathology of dementia, the aim here is to give an outline of what is known rather than a comprehensive presentation. For a more detailed examination of the epidemiology of dementia the reader is referred to Bergmann (1969), Slater and Roth (1969), or Pearce and Miller (1973). Nevertheless the discussion of epidemiology will not be quite as cursory as that of pathology since this is the only place in which epidemiological factors will be dealt with and some issues relating to the pathology of dementia will emerge in later chapters.

Present knowledge about the epidemiology of dementia in the presenile age range is very sparse. One of the very few relevant publications is that of Sjogren et al. (1952). Sjogren examined the records of psychiatric hospitals in and around the Swedish cities of Gothenburg and Stockholm for cases of Pick's and Alzheimer's diseases over two decades. From this data he was able to estimate that the morbidity risk for Alzheimer's and Pick's diseases combined was 0·1%. This is much less than the morbidity risk of 1% which the same author had previously established for senile dementia. The average age of onset for both Alzheimer's and Pick's diseases was in the mid-fifties with the mean time from onset of the illness to death being 7 years. This means that the life expectancy of a case of presenile dementia of these types is less than half that of a normal person of the same age.

Sjogren found an appreciably increased morbidity risk for dementia in the relatives of his probands. The data was not extensive enough to justify any firm conclusions about possible mechanisms of inheritance but Sjogren felt that it pointed towards a multifactorial inheritance in Alzheimer's disease and a dominant inheritance with modifying genes for Pick's disease. An interesting feature of Sjogren's series is that all the cases for whom there were full pathological studies after death, in the Gothenburg hospitals, were cases of Alzheimer's disease. In the Stockholm hospitals there was a heavy preponderance of Pick's disease in those cases subjected to the same detailed investigations.

It is fortunate that the epidemiology of dementia in the senile age range has been much more extensively studied. Estimates of the prevalence of dementia (including cases assumed to be arteriosclerotic in aetiology) vary between about 5% and 15% of the elderly population (see Slater and Roth, 1969). The discrepancies between the various sets of figures can be at least partly explained by differences in the criteria used to identify probands. In Britain the most extensive studies have been carried out by Roth and his associates in Newcastle-upon-Tyne. In a detailed survey of elderly subjects living at home and in institutions, Kay et al. (1964a) found an overall prevalence of about 10% for senile and arteriosclerotic dementia combined. Of this 10% about half were judged to have severe or moderate mental deterioration and the rest had a mild degree of mental deterioration. Arteriosclerotic brain syndromes were judged to be more common in males and senile dementia more prevalent in females. An interesting point is that 5% of the elderly living at home had dementia as severe as that occurring in hospitalized subjects, a finding that might partly reflect the importance of social factors in determining admission to hospital or other types of institution.

The prevalence of dementia increases with age. Kay et al. (1970) examined a further sample of elderly subjects in Newcastle-upon-Tyne. More-stringent

TABLE 2
Prevalence of 'chronic brain syndrome'
(i.e., dementia) in Newcastle-upon-
Tyne. Data taken from Kay *et al.*
(1970)

Age (years)	Prevalence (%)
65–69	2·3
70–74	2·8
75–79	5·5
80 and over	22·0
Total	6·2

criteria of dementia were used and the new data from this survey was combined with that from the previous survey after excluding from the latter those cases that did not meet the stricter criteria of the later study. This reduced the overall prevalence rate for those over 65 years to 6·2%. The very large sample obtained in this way enabled prevalence rates to be estimated for different age groups and these are given in Table 2. It can be seen that the prevalence rate increases dramatically for subjects over 80 years old.

Senile dementia, like the presenile forms, results in a very much reduced life expectancy. Roth (1955) showed that elderly patients with dementia in a psychiatric hospital had a very much higher mortality rate than those of a similar age with functional psychiatric disorders. Kay (1962) observed that the mean length of survival of patients admitted to a Swedish psychiatric hospital and suffering from senile dementia was 2½ years. Not only does the demented patient have a shorter life expectancy but his demands upon hospital services are very much increased. Kay *et al.* (1970) estimated that demented subjects were three times as likely as psychiatrically normal subjects to be admitted to hospitals and clinics of *all* types including those dealing with physical diseases.

As far as genetic aspects are concerned it is well established that the relatives of patients with senile dementia have an increased morbidity risk. Despite at least one large scale investigation, the actual mode of inheritance is unclear. Larsson *et al.* (1963) came down in favour of a single autosomal dominant gene but other authorities have favoured recessive or multifactorial inheritance (Bergmann, 1969).

Of greater possible interest in the present context is the relationship between dementia and social factors. A characteristic of elderly demented subjects is that they tend to be socially isolated as compared with other old people. This finding has emerged in a number of reports (Fisch *et al.*, 1968; Garside *et al.*, 1965; and Larsson *et al.*, (1963) but the relationship between dementia and social isolation is not a simple one. Demented subjects are prone to physical and sensory handicaps (Kay *et al.*, 1964b) and these are likely to cause or contribute to social isolation. Garside *et al.* (1965) found that bereavement, which must be an important factor in causing social isolation in the elderly, was not related to dementia. These authors rightly comment that social isolation is a complex variable which may need further refinement or subdivision before it is of real use.

There is little evidence that dementia is related to socioeconomic status. The only influence of social class which emerged in the extensive investigations of Larsson *et al.* (1963) was in the case of single females with dementia who were on average of lower socioeconomic status. Whilst social class is probably not related to the incidence of dementia it may well have a bearing on what happens to the individual once the illness has got under way. American studies (see Fisch *et al.*, 1968) have shown that factors involved in low social status, such as a low level of education and low income, are associated with hospitalization for all psychiatric diseases of the senium.

Kay *et al.* (1964b) have discussed the possible mechanisms which might relate social factors to dementia. They point out that these cannot be considered to be primary causes of dementia and are often more probably the consequence of the illness. In a few cases social isolation could contribute to the progression of an already established dementing illness by enhancing the depression that is found in many cases. Depression can lead to self-neglect with dietary deficiencies which could then assist the dementing process.

SOME OTHER PRELIMINARY ISSUES

The following chapters will give, firstly, an outline of the psychological changes that occur as a result of normal ageing and will then go on to deal with the various psychological aspects of abnormal ageing, or dementia, in some detail. Before proceeding with this plan some preliminary issues need to be discussed.

It has become increasingly fashionable amongst psychologists interested in abnormal behaviour to reject the usual psychiatric nosology as a basis for their work (e.g., Costello, 1970; Eysenck, 1960). This dissatisfaction has started with the extensive evidence indicating that the conventional psychiatric diagnoses generally have low reliability. It has gained further momentum from the desire to set aside the so-called 'medical model' of mental illness and to substitute social or psychological models. Undoubtedly this has become something of a bandwagon in which some of the advocates of change have not really thought their arguments through and thus appear to be jumping out of the medical frying pan into a social sciences fire. Nevertheless, in many aspects of abnormal psychology there is a great deal in favour of the move away from medical diagnoses as a basis for study and a move towards those, like Costello (1970), who favour the analysis of symptoms rather than syndromes.

Within the area of concern of the present work, the principal exponent of an approach which rejects medical diagnosis has been Inglis. In his many experiments concerned with memory processes in elderly subjects, he has stressed that he is dealing with elderly psychiatric patients who have memory disorders (e.g., Inglis, 1960) and not patients who have dementia. In practice Inglis (1970) admits that his elderly 'memory disordered' subjects would have the label 'senile dementia' attached to them and in describing Inglis' experimental work later in Chapter Four, the assumption will be made that 'memory disordered' is synonymous with 'dementia'. Whilst it is the case that memory disorder can occur in old age without being due to dementia, such cases are very rare and as a result the assumption of identity is not likely to give rise to much error.

The rejection of the diagnosis of dementia as a basis for study runs counter to the whole approach in this book and it is now necessary to defend the retention of the diagnostic label. As indicated above there are two main reasons for rejecting the diagnosis of dementia in psychological investigations. These are that the diagnosis cannot be made with sufficient accuracy and that it implies an inappropriate model for the problem. To take the latter point first, there is no serious argument that dementia does not have a physical basis. Therefore, the 'medical model' is appropriate although it must be added that this does not imply that the psychological manifestations of the disease are not important. Providing that care is taken in the original evaluation, a diagnosis of dementia can be made with reasonable accuracy. Because few other conditions have the same poor prognosis as dementia with its gradual deterioration, follow up of subjects for a short period can confirm the diagnosis. As a result it is held that dementia is a diagnosis that provides a viable basis for psychological study but this is not to uphold all psychiatric diagnostic categories, particularly those relating to the functional disorders, in the same way.

Unfortunately it does not mean that because the diagnosis of dementia can be accomplished with accuracy everyone who uses the term will have been equally careful in establishing the diagnosis, or that some small differences might not emerge in comparing different experimental reports because of the use of slightly different diagnostic criteria. Those authors presenting investigations carried out on patients in psychiatric hospitals are likely to be dealing with more advanced cases than, say, the present writer who always uses presenile cases in the early stages undergoing investigations in a neurological unit. Demonstration of cerebral atrophy by air encephalography is much more likely to have been carried out in patients investigated in a neurological unit and detailed investigations of this type are usually only considered justified in the younger demented patient. In institutions where it has incorrectly been assumed that all dementias without demonstrable cause are due to cerebral arteriosclerosis, it is most unlikely that those cases with positive indications of arteriosclerosis will have been separated out.

Despite these problems, which may require some minor modification of opinions when fully resolved, it is possible to make a reasonable review of the psychology of dementia based on the evidence available at present. This is particularly worthwhile because in the present state of knowledge the problem of dementia is that of its management. The consideration of management in turn brings us face to face with the question of the way in which the patient with dementia functions.

2
Normal Ageing

Dementia is a condition that is found in the older individual and the effects of dementia must be considered against the background of normal ageing. The psychological and other features in dementia will be a compound of the effects of the disease process and changes which would have occurred anyway as a result of the normal processes of ageing. For this reason it is appropriate to have some idea of the psychological changes associated with normal ageing before passing on to the consequences of dementia.

This chapter will give a brief outline of the psychology of normal ageing. Because normal ageing is a very large topic in itself, this chapter can only give a limited presentation of the basic problems and findings. It is in no way intended to compete with the standard works on the psychology of ageing or to give an up-to-the-minute review of recent research trends and controversies. The main reason for writing this chapter is merely to give a minimum background in normal ageing to those readers who come to this book with a largely clinical background and who may need a reminder about normal processes. Those familiar with the literature on the psychology of normal ageing might prefer to go straight on to Chapter 3.

GENERAL CONSIDERATIONS

Like many concepts in everyday use, that of 'ageing' causes no problems in common usage but ceases to be quite so simple and straightforward when subjected to detailed scrutiny (see Bromley, 1974, for a more detailed exposition of the issues involved.) In normal usage we do not distinguish the mere passage of time from the changes that occur within time when we talk of 'ageing'. Time is neutral in that it cannot produce any effect by itself, it is the factors that operate within time which produce any change that occurs.

One way of dealing with this situation is to distinguish between 'chronological age', as marked by the passage of time, and 'functional age'. As far as any function is concerned, whether it be physical like the basal metabolic rate, or psychological like reaction time, an individual of, say, 60 years may function like the average subject of a rather higher or lower chronological age. This functional age is therefore a concept rather akin to 'mental age' and will share many of the well known methodological difficulties of the latter. One particular problem with functional age is that different functions within the same individual do not necessarily change in step with one another. An extreme example is the young adult male who shows appreciable baldness well before he is 30 and yet functions as a young adult in all other ways. For this reason it is most unlikely that it will ever be possible to allot an overall functional age to any individual.

A further problem with the concept of ageing (or rather the changes that occur with ageing) is the extent to which it is presumed to reflect some form of underlying general process. Such an underlying process is to some extent generally assumed by the current interest in 'lifespan developmental psychology' which has the laudable aim of trying to set human development and ageing within a single continuous framework (e.g., Goulet and Baltes, 1970). Bromley (1972) illustrates one of his discussions of this point by using an apt military analogy. If a battle is considered, the army that wins convincingly can be described as having followed a directed process even though there may well have been some deviation from the general's plan. However, the army in opposition that was routed does not display a similar direction in its panic and flight from the field. As Bromley points out, early development seems to be a directed process in a similar sense to the victory being a directed process but the processes of ageing may well prove to be more like the rout in having no overall direction.

The study of ageing also raises important methodological issues. These will be given the briefest airing at this point because the next section on the intellectual changes associated with ageing will provide a good concrete illustration of some of the major points. At its simplest there are two different research strategies. The first, and most commonly used because it is the easiest, is the cross-sectional study. This is based on the comparison of separate groups of subjects at different age levels. A likely source of bias in this method is that the patterns of upbringing, educational opportunity, etc. are constantly changing and so the younger and older groups may not be comparable with regard to important environmental influences. Bias may also be introduced into the older groups because some types of subjects may tend to survive longer than others and will then tend to overpredominate in the older groups when samples are drawn.

The alternative technique is the longitudinal study in which the same sample is followed over an appreciable amount of their life span. The problems are obvious. It is difficult to keep track of subjects over relatively short periods of time and the task of doing so is formidable when the period involved is likely to be of the order of decades. Such studies have to go on for a considerable length of time before they yield useful data and they may even exceed the lifespan of the original investigator! At a more technical level there are also complications raised by the repeated use of many psychological measures (e.g., practice effects).

As we shall see in the next section, a combination of the cross-sectional and longitudinal techniques can be used to good effect (Schiae and Strother, 1968a). This involves the follow-up of cross-sectional samples for a relatively short period. Nevertheless this still leaves some methodological problems that are common to all research strategies. There is good reason to believe that the same procedure applied to both young and old subjects may not always be measuring quite the same thing within the two samples (e.g., Gilmore, 1972).

A final important consideration in studies of ageing, which has already been adumbrated in the opening paragraphs of this book, is that the factors underlying age-related changes are extremely complex. It can be very unwise to take an age-related change on any psychological variable and simply assume that the older person differs from the younger on the basis of that particular variable. Older people are much more prone to sensory defects and to a wide range of diseases and both these things can affect functional capacity. To take a single example, hypertension is much more common in older people and Wilkie and Eisdorfer (1971) have found that hypertension is associated with lower intelligence test performance.

Some attempt can be made to control for physical changes known to affect performance although this is rarely done in practice. Of at least equal importance and rather more difficult to deal with are the motivational, attitudinal and social changes. The older person may be less well motivated or have a less tolerant attitude towards the rather strange things that the research psychologist requires him to do. The general social ethos of old age as a time of rest and quiet enjoyment is probably not compatible with the almost competitive nature of many experimental tasks, e.g. those involved in the measure of reaction times. Factors of this type can be important sources of variation in experiments on ageing but the rather doubtful assertion that they can provide a total explanation for age-related psychological deficits will be discussed later.

The multiplicity of factors underlying age changes also indicates that the psychological aspects, here considered in isolation, are but one facet of the whole. Gerontology is a multidisciplinary subject and failure to take other aspects into account is liable to lead the study of the psychology of ageing into difficulties.

INTELLIGENCE AND AGEING

It is commonly accepted that abilities increase throughout childhood and reach a peak in early adult life. There is then a decline, slow at first, but accelerating in later life. This relationship between ability and age is illustrated in Figure 1 which is based on Wechsler's (1955) standardization data for his Adult Intelligence Scale. This sort of picture of the decline of intellectual abilities with age has been widely cited in the past. It has been used to back up claims of the kind that older individuals are much less capable of being trained in new jobs. In more recent times extensive evidence has appeared to suggest that this picture may not be accurate at least as far as intelligence is concerned.

The pattern of decline with increasing age shown in Figure 1, and other illustrations of this type, is in fact based on cross-sectional data in that the various points on the curve come from averaging the results of samples of different age levels. The implicit assumption is that the only relevant variable

15

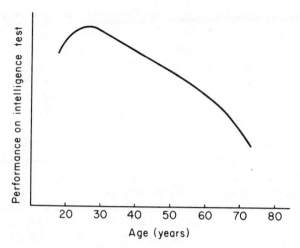

Figure 1. Intelligence test performance as a function of age. Based on data extracted from Wechsler (1955)

distinguishing between samples at different age levels is their age. Educational opportunities and nutritional standards have improved quite markedly in Western countries during this century and in particular between the dates of birth of the oldest and youngest subjects used in the samples. It is well established that both these factors can affect performance in intelligence tests (e.g., Husen, 1951). The result is likely to be a bias in favour of the younger subjects and hence the extent of any intellectual decline with age will be exaggerated.

A longitudinal study over the whold of the subjects' adult lifespans might give a better picture but there is no such report in the literature. Even a longitudinal study of this type might not give a completely accurate picture because scores on intelligence tests, like those of the commonly used Wechsler series, do change as a result of retesting (e.g., Matarazzo, *et al.*, 1973) and there is no guarantee that the inevitable attrition in the sample over time by death, disease, or simply failure to trace, would not introduce biases. What is available is a small number of reports of the results of retesting adult groups a considerable number of years after the initial tests. In general these support the idea that curves like that given in Figure 1 do overestimate the rate of decline with age. Owens (1966) had 96 male subjects tested on the Army Alpha test at around the age of 50 and again 11 years later. There was only a slight trend to lower scores but it was nowhere near statistical significance.

Of particular interest is a much more sophisticated investigation by Schaie and Strother (1968a; 1968b). They had several separate samples of subjects drawn in a cross-sectional manner at each 5-year age interval from 20 to 70 years. Subjects were tested on the primary Mental Abilities test and each subject was retested 7 years later. This experimental design is a mixture of both cross-sectional and longitudinal methods and permits a comparison between the two. Their pattern of results confirmed that cross-sectional data overestimated age changes except where speed was a very important factor in test performance.

It is probably safe to conclude that, whilst intellectual performance does decline with age and most markedly at older age levels, this deterioration in performance is not as drastic as had once been supposed. Another problem apart from the rate at which intellectual decline occurs comes from the fact that intelligence test scores are global measures covering a large number of more specific abilities. Are some types of intellectual ability more liable to decline with age and, if so, how can we describe the pattern of change?

We have already seen that Schaie and Strother (1968b) have reported that tests which have a strong speed component are especially likely to show marked deterioration with age. Slowing is a generally accepted feature of ageing and will emerge in other contexts within this chapter. The normative data on the Wechsler Adult Intelligence Scale shows that some subtests are more susceptible to decline with age than others (Wechsler, 1958). It is difficult to specify a common characteristic of the subtests like Digit Symbol and Block Design which tend to show large age-related changes as opposed to Vocabulary and other subtests which do not. One feature of possible importance is that the subtests showing most change seem to involve memory or the ability to adduce new relationships, whilst those at the other end of the scale are more concerned with acquired knowledge. Wechsler has tried to make use of this differential decline in subtests to devise a 'deterioration index' for measuring intellectual decline in individual subjects. This involves the comparison of scores on four 'hold' tests (Vocabulary, Object Assembly, Information, and Picture Completion) with four 'don't hold' tests (Digit Span, Similarities, Digit Symbol, and Block Design). The clinical use of the Wechsler Deterioration Index will be discussed in Chapter 8.

Schaie and Strother (1968b) also found that some subtests of the Primary Mental Abilities held up better than others. The longitudinal aspect of their study showed that Verbal Meaning, Number, Space and Reasoning only started to show appreciable decline in the early sixties. Word Fluency, a test with a very strong speed component started to decline much earlier. Schaie and Gribbin (1975) also argue that the point at which decline starts to be manifest is moving up the age scale with succeeding generations. Just why this should be happening and whether it will tend to decrease or exaggerate the difference in rate of decline between different tests is not discussed.

Others have attempted to characterize the decline produced by ageing in more general terms. Goldstein and Scheerer (1941) distinguished between the abstract and concrete attitudes in thinking. This distinction was originally introduced to describe the effects of brain damage on thought processes but it has been applied more widely both to schizophrenic thought disorder and to the effects of normal ageing. Abstract and concrete thinking is usually examined by means of sorting tests and Thaler (1956) has obtained results which could be interpreted as showing more concrete behaviour in older subjects.

A different subdivision of intellectual skills has been proposed by Cattell

(1943) and developed by him in later publications. Briefly Cattell proposes a 'fluid' intelligence which relates more to the potential of the individual to acquire new ideas and to adapt to new situations. There is also a 'crystallized' intelligence which largely consists of learned intellectual skills. Thus learning to solve, say, a particular type of differential equation will require fluid intelligence, but, once this skill has been mastered, it becomes crystallized. The suggestion has been that fluid ability declines more rapidly with age than crystallized abilities.

Much of the data on intellectual changes in ageing could be considered to be consistent with this notion (see Savage, 1973 for a much fuller review) and so is the brief comment above regarding the differential decline in the Wechsler subtests. Amongst the large number of examples that might be cited here is an investigation by Cunningham *et al.* (1975), which is also of interest because it shows one possible way round some of the major methodological problems of research on ageing. Cunningham *et al.* predicted, on the basis of the notion that fluid intelligence deteriorates more rapidly than does crystallized intelligence, that correlations between measures of these two types of intelligence would be higher in young adults than in a sample of elderly subjects. Since this prediction says nothing about the relative amounts of change or when that change starts to occur, the awkward pitfalls of the usual cross-sectional design are avoided. Using the Raven's Progressive Matrices and the Wechsler Vocabulary Scale as the measures of fluid and crystallized intelligence respectively these authors were able to confirm the prediction with two samples of different age levels.

The distinction between fluid and crystallized abilities has a number of parallels with other very general theoretical distinctions in intelligence like Hebb's (1949) discussion of 'Intellegence A' and 'Intelligence B'. Since such distinctions are at a level far removed from the behaviour of subjects on specific tests it is easy to get evidence which generally supports the low-level predictions that these 'theories' generate.

What is required are some alternative approaches to the study of intelligence as it changes with ageing. Some alternatives have been discussed by Bromley (1972) but will not be elaborated here because they have not yet been extensively exploited in the study of normal ageing and have certainly not percolated through to the study of abnormal ageing. One line of work that particularly merits a brief comment is the use of Piagetian techniques. Although Piaget has been concerned almost exclusively with the development of intellectual abilities, it is possible to take his ideas and techniques and apply them to the study of the ways in which intellectual abilities break down. So far the small amount of Piagetian research on ageing seems to suffer from poor methodology. Storck *et al.* (1972) looked at the performance of a group of older adult subjects (aged 55 to 79 years) in tests of concrete operational thought (e.g., weight conservation) and tests of formal operational thought (e.g., volume conservation). Their subjects did well on the tests of concrete operations but much less well on the tests of formal operations. However, this finding only makes sense as showing a deterioration in the level of intellectual functioning that can be achieved if it is also assumed that young adults would have performed satisfactorily on the tests of formal operations.

OTHER ASPECTS OF COGNITIVE FUNCTIONING

There are other ways of looking at intellectual functioning besides using the usual tests of 'intelligence'. There is therefore a great deal that could be subsumed under this heading but a few illustrative studies will have to suffice. Although the investigations to be described fall within a number of different traditions within psychology, all agree in suggesting that older people are particularly impaired in certain specific types of intellectual activity.

In a series of sorting experiments, Rabbitt (1965) had decks of cards with each card having one or more letters on it although the cards in any one deck contained the same number of letters. Each card contained an 'A' or a 'B' randomly situated amongst the other letters (which were not As or Bs) if such were present in a particular pack. The subject's task was to sort the cards into piles according to whether the card contained an 'A' or a 'B'. In comparing old and young adults on this and similar tasks it was found that not only were the older subjects slower but that the addition of irrelevant information in the shape of the extra letters had a much more deleterious effect on the speed of sorting of the older subjects. This reduced ability of the older subject to ignore irrelevant information could have wide ranging implications if it is found to generalize to other tasks. This is because many everyday tasks present the subject with a large amount of information much of which is irrelevant and has to be ignored.

By contrast, Wetherick (1966) examined concept formation in older people using a task based on those described by Bruner *et al.* (1956). The basic idea of the experimental technique is to have a population of stimuli which can vary along a number of different dimensions (in this case letters of the alphabet in different positions on cards). The subject is shown a series of examples, one at a time, which illustrate or do not illustrate a particular concept (e.g., a word containing both an 'A' and a 'B'). He is told whether or not each example is an example of the concept and then has to state what he thinks the concept is. By carefully selecting the examples and the order in which they are presented and then analysing the errors it is possible to gain an indication as to why the subject failed to discern the concept. Wetherick found that older subjects tended to make errors indicating the application of inappropriate strategies and especially by treating a negative instance as if it were a positive one. There was also a slight trend towards older subjects being less likely to make an error based on a failure to take account of all the available information.

It is difficult to leave this area without mentioning Lehman's classical studies of achievement (Lehman, 1953; 1962, 1964). Lehman's general technique is to take the members of a particular academic or professional group (e.g., chemists or engineers) and to look at their significant contributions as a function of age. The common finding for both pure and applied scientists is that their published contributions begin in their early twenties and rise steeply to a maximum in the middle thirties and decline. The actual peak age varies a little from group to group. Other aspects of human endeavour do not show quite this pattern. In musical composition, for example, maximum productivity is also reached in the mid-thirties but productivity remains a high level until old age is reached.

Without going into Lehman's extensive studies in any detail, it is roughly true to say that intellectual productivity, especially of a scientific nature, is usually maximal in the thirties. At first sight this seems strong evidence in support of the picture of intellectual change given by cross-sectional studies with a relatively early decline in ability. However, certain reservations must be entered in addition to the fact that the sort of people who make the kind of major contributions that Lehman looked at are not representative of the general population. As scientists become more eminent they become more involved in administrative work and more sought after as speakers at conferences and members of government commissions. Not only does the middle-aged distingui-shed scientist have less time for original work but he begins to suffer another disadvantage with respect to his younger colleagues. The younger scientist's training is closer to the current state of knowledge in his discipline and he therefore has less in the way of superceded information to unlearn. These factors in no way diminish the possibility that the sorts of abilities necessary for making important original contributions to science might decline more quickly than many other abilities with age, they merely cast doubt on the particular time scale given by Lehman.

MEMORY AND LEARNING

The study of learning and memory in humans has followed a number of traditions. Following on the paths of Ebbinghaus have been those who have been almost exclusively concerned with the acquisition and retention of verbal materials; lists of nonsense syllables, paired associate learning, and the like. Others have studied such things as simple conditioning, using what could be considered as human analogues of animal experiments, and the learning of motor skills usually without reference to verbal learning. For this reason it is convenient to divide this brief review of learning and memory in ageing into two separate parts, dealing first with verbal memory and then with the remaining aspects of learning and memory.

A further complicating factor in the study of learning and memory is that the processes involved are quite complex. New information has to be acquired, held in storage and then retrieved when necessary. Any decline with ageing could be due to a failure in any of these stages and many experimental psycho-logists would wish to subdivide the process even further, e.g. the distinction between short-term and long-term storage. In fact much of the work on verbal memory, which we will consider first, has been carried out in an attempt to decide which aspects of the total process are particularly likely to deteriorate with ageing.

This is no simple task and it is easy to reach the wrong conclusions because of accidental factors in the experimental design. Gilbert and Levee (1971) tried a 'blunderbuss' approach by giving the Guild Memory Test to normal subjects between the ages of 35 and 75 years. This test has subtests which purport to measure different aspects of the memory processes and Gilbert and Levee found that some subtests showed much more decline than others. Leaving aside the question of the validity of the subtests, it is difficult to get a sensible answer by having just one test for each aspect of memory. These may reveal that acquisition of new material is poor in the older subject but that retrieval information from storage survives relatively well. However, an acquisition test using a slower rate of presentation of material, and hence making acquisition easier for all subjects, may give no age differences and a more searching test of recall may show deficits in retrieval. For this reason the different aspects of memory need to be considered separately and in depth.

A common explanation of the lowered ability of the elderly to learn and/or retain information has been that the acquisition of new material is particularly prone to deterioration and, more specifically, that short-term memory is reduced. Inglis et al. (1968) have described a series of experiments using Broadbent's (1954) dichotic listening technique. In general it was found that older subjects were impaired when it came to reporting stimuli from the second ear. Since in this type of experiment the subject hears stimuli simultaneously in both ears but reports all those to one ear first, it follows that the stimuli presented to the second ear must be maintained for a short period in some form of temporary storage which Inglis equates with short-term memory. A number of other investigators, using rather different experimental techniques, have also obtained results consistent with the hypothesis that short-term memory is affected (e.g., Kinsbourne, 1973; McGhie et al., 1965, and Taub, 1975). On the other hand there have been a few negative findings (e.g., Craik, 1968, and Drachman and Leavitt, 1972).

Factors have been identified which sometimes seem to differentiate the performance of older and younger subjects on tasks related to short-term memory. In Kinsbourne's (1973) experiment, subjects' ability to recall short letter sequences was considered as a function of rate of presentation as well as of age. The rate of presentation of letters was varied between one letter every 2 seconds to four letters per second which is quite a wide range. As well as giving a lower overall level of performance the elderly group found the faster presentation rates much more difficult whilst the young adults were unaffected by the rate of presentation. The same experiment also showed that altering the sequential probabilities of the letter sequences to being more in line with the normal letter sequences in English helped both groups equally, thus showing that the elderly still retain their ability to make use of redundancy.

The modality in which the material has been presented has also been considered to be of importance in experiments on short-term memory. McGhie *et al.* (1965) and others have observed that performance declines more rapidly when the material is presented in the visual modality than when it is presented in the auditory modality. This makes some sense in terms of what is known about coding in short-term memory. Somehow incoming material must be transformed or coded in order to be stored and there is evidence (e.g., Baddeley, 1966a) that verbal material in short-term memory is coded by its auditory characteristics irrespective of the modality of presentation. Where incoming information is in the visual modality it will have to be translated into an auditory form before it can be stored in short-term memory and a reduced ability to make this type of transformation could be an important part of the memory deficit in ageing (Marcer, 1974). Unfortunately for this line of reasoning, Taub (1975) has recently pointed to some methodological inadequacies in the key experiments. On reexamining this question he was unable to replicate the finding that the older subject is more prone to show decline in short-term memory with visual presentation although, given comparable material, both old and young found auditory presentation easier than visual.

A final problem with these studies of short-term memory is that any loss of capacity in short-term memory might be, at least partly, an artifact. Experimental procedures purporting to be concerned with short-term memory usually measure output from short-term memory. Output may be reduced because short-term memory is impaired or because information fails to reach short-term memory adequately because of deficits in attention, perception, or even 'iconic memory' (Neisser, 1967). Kline and Szafran (1975) showed that tachistoscopically-presented digits were more vulnerable to the effects of backward masking by a following 'visual noise' field in older subjects. This could be explained by a more rapid rate of decay in iconic memory in older subjects. Similarly with the auditory modality, Clark and Knowles (1973) have reexamined the dichotic listening situation used by Inglis and his associates. Clark and Knowles carried out a more complicated version of the dichotic listening experiment in which they varied the order of report of each ear, and the method of report, in order to see whether age changes were the result of registration, retention or retrieval deficits. They concluded that the main problem for the older subject was in the initial perception or registration of information rather than in retention or retrieval. Of course neither of these experiments prove that short-term memory as such is not affected, but they do suggest that at least part of the problem lies in the earlier stage of registration of stimuli.

Other aspects of the total memory process are also of concern. Some have contended that long-term storage and retrieval remain intact with ageing but their experimental evidence is not always convincing. Moenster (1972) required her subjects to listen to a story and answer questions about it immediately afterwards and then some time later. She found that tests of both immediate and later retention declined with age but an analysis of convariance to control for immediate retention eliminated the decline with age on the later retention scores. She argued that the immediate testing reflected learning, and when this was taken into account the age differences disappeared, so the effect of age must be solely on learning. Unfortunately this interpretation is unjustified. The story was long enough to exceed the usual estimates of normal short-term memory capacity many times over and therefore any recall of more than a very few items at the immediate test must, of necessity, have involved information that had been passed through to, and retrieved from, long-term memory. On the basis of this argument Moenster's experiment is merely giving us the not unexpected finding that the amount of information entering long-term memory accounts for most of the variance in later recall.

Evidence strongly suggestive of impairments in long-term storage or retrieval comes from a number of sources. Laurence (1967) had subjects listen to a single presentation of a list of 36 words. Equal numbers of words fell into one of six categories (names of flowers, birds, etc.) and subjects were given the names of these categories either at the time of presentation or at the time of recall. Being given this cue at the time of presentation had no effect on the recall of either group but it did improve the performance of the older subjects when given at the time of recall. This was to such a degree that older group's recall equalled that of the younger.

If giving the appropriate cue (category names in this instance) can enhance the older subjects recall to a level equivalent to that of the young adult, it follows that the information (at least under the particular presentation conditions used) must originally have been acquired with the same facility and that the older person's difficulty must lie at the point of retrieval. Unfortunately retrieval processes in the elderly have not been as widely explored as the acquisition of new information, although there are others (e.g., Schonfield, 1967; Smith, 1975) who have presented arguments for the importance of factors operating in long-term memory and especially at the time of retrieval. Smith used a paired-associate learning paradigm to explore the effect of interference in age-related memory changes. His main hypothesis, that the elderly were more prone to interference, was not confirmed but the pattern of results indicated that it was long-term rather than short-term memory that was primarily affected.

Of the large number of other issues in the general field of verbal learning and memory that have been raised in the literature, space only permits the brief mention of a small sample. There have been suggestions (e.g., Schonfield and Robertson, 1966) that recognition memory is not affected by ageing, unlike recall. Erber (1974) claims that this may be because the recognition tests used were not sensitive enough and his own results support this contention. Eysenck (1975), using matched recall and recognition tasks, found that recognition could even be more impaired than recall under some circumstances.

One possible explanation of poorer memory in older persons is that they are more prone to interference. Smith (1975) found that paired-associate learning in the elderly was no more or less prone to the effects of proactive and retroactive interference, but Boyarsky and Eisdorfer's (1972) older group were more liable to interference from contextual associations on a modified free recall task. As a final point, Gordon and Clark (1974) used a signal detection theory approach to memory changes and produced evidence that the reduced ability to retain material in the elderly was due to a definite loss of ability to discriminate between previously learned information and presented alternatives, and not to an alteration in the response criterion. One important implication of this experiment is that it shows the memory disturbance with ageing to be real and not an artifact produced by, say, poor motivation in the elderly.

We shall now pass to a consideration of 'non-verbal' aspects of memory and learning. (The term 'non-verbal' of course only refers to the skills or materials to be learned since subjects may well use verbal mediation in a task that is not overtly verbal.) Since the work to be dealt with in abnormal ageing contains relatively little on non-verbal aspects of leaning, the topic will only be treated rather cursorily with regard to normal ageing.

With reference to studies of simple conditioning, there are reports that the elderly are slow to learn on a classical eye-blink conditioning task (Braun and Geiselhart, 1959; Kimble and Pennybacker, 1963). Botwinick and Kornetsky (1960) used the classical conditioning of the galvanic skin response and found that the elderly were quicker to extinguish as well as being slower to learn. The results of all these studies are consistent with Botwinick and Kornetsky's explanation of the changes in terms of the older subjects' lower reactivity.

An area of special interest within the study of learning in relation to age is the ability of the older person to learn new skills. This is of some social importance because increasing automation and changes in the pattern of industrial manpower needs mean that many middle age workers become redundant. Their potential for retraining has rightly been of concern to psychologists in the field of ageing. The common prejudice that the older worker cannot learn new skills has not been supported. Those apparent deficits that have emerged are small and have sometimes been shown to be, at least partly, the consequence of other factors than poor learning *per se* (Birren, 1964). Furthermore, experiments like those of Belbin (1958) and Belbin and Downs (1964) demonstrate that some of the relative slowness of the older workers in the acquisition of new skills can be compensated for by the use of appropriate training methods. It should also be remembered that the work on industrial skills has been concerned with the older people within the normal working age range and not the elderly persons of above retirement age to which the rest of the work on ageing generally refers.

PERSONALITY

There is a certain amount of folk wisdom regarding personality changes with age. Generally older people are considered to be more set in their ways and to hold more rigidly to their beliefs and opinions. The characteristic traits of the ageing individual are believed to change. The older person may be considered to mellow and prominent traits are reduced in intensity; drive and ambition decline. Alternatively some of the less desirable features of personality, such as irritability, may become exaggerated.

The objective assessment of personality changes due to ageing presents methodological problems additional to those encountered in other areas of ageing. As well as the usual technical problems involved in the measurement of personality there is the very real possibility that personality questionnaires may not be measuring the same things at different ages. Gilmore (1972) has noted that questionnaire items may not be understood by the elderly, or may be understood in a way that is different from the meaning attributed to them by the younger subjects on whom the test was developed.

The typical finding when old and young subjects are compared on the standard personality questionnaires is that the personality profiles tend to be very much the same. Some consistent changes are found but these are not very marked. When Hardyck (1964) compared younger with older women on the Minnesota Multiphasic Personality Inventory, it was observed that the elderly had higher scores on the hysteria and hypochondriasis scales. It could be argued that the change towards increased hypochondriasis might be justified by the older person's greater susceptibility to disease. The older subjects also showed lower levels of hypomania, a finding in accord with clinical evidence of age changes in the incidence of hypomania, and a trend towards more conservative attitudes. These results are similar to those reported previously by Brozek (1955) who applied the same personality inventory to men. In a fairly recent review Schaie and Marquette (1972) list introversion, cautiousness, lower responsivity, lower needs for achievement, lower heterosexuality and fewer signs of psychopathology as being related to increasing age.

Two generally acknowledged personality characteristics of the aged are particularly singled out by Botwinick (1973) in his general review of psychological aspects of ageing. These are cautiousness and rigidity. As Botwinick clearly points out, and despite the common use of these terms to characterize the behaviour of the elderly, neither of them is a unitary concept and the evidence indicates that there is no single trait of cautiousness or rigidity. In her work on rigidity, Chown (1960, 1962) has concluded that there are many different types of rigidity and that much of what is usually considered to come under the heading of 'rigidity' may be produced by intellectual decline. It is quite reasonable to suppose that the intellectual decline in old age with its reduced ability to handle the complexities of situations will result in a more stereotyped and rigid way of dealing with new problems.

Botwinick (1973) cites a large amount of evidence which might be interpreted as showing increased cautiousness in the elderly, e.g. in needing to be more sure of the correctness of a response before they would respond in an experimental task. In one of his own experiments, Botwinick (1966) asked his subjects to give advice to a young person facing a series of fictional life situations. Older subjects were usually more inclined to 'play safe' and not advise a risky course of Action. As with rigidity, there is also evidence that cautiousness may be secondary to other factors. Edwards and Vine (1963) used both an intelligence test and a personality measure of cautiousness. When the older subjects were matched with the younger for scores on the intelligence test the trend for cautiousness to increase with age was eliminated.

Interests also change with age and one very frequently cited study is that of Pressey and Kuhlen (1957). These authors analysed responses to the Strong Vocational Interest Blank and showed that older persons had a decline in active interests (e.g., sport and politics). There was a corresponding increase in more solitary and sedentary pursuits such as gardening and bird watching. These results are quite consistent with the more sociologically-based descriptions of the changes produced by ageing as being those of withdrawal and social disengagement.

It would be inappropriate to leave the topic of personality and related functions without some mention of disengagement theory. This was first proposed by Cumming and Henry (1961) but subsequent modifications have become necessary and convenient summaries can be found in Botwinick, (1973), Bromley (1974) and Neugarten (1973). It is a well attested observation that as people grow older their activities becomes curtailed. The more traditional view has been that the elderly have similar psychological and social needs to those which they had in middle age and that the decreased social involvement in old age is primarily the result of society withdrawing from the elderly. Cumming and Henry differed in that they regard the withdrawal as mutual or even initiated by the elderly person himself. It is not that society excludes him but that he is active in excluding himself. The corollary of this theory is that the older person who has successfully withdrawn will be better adjusted and have a higher satisfaction with life. If the alternative view is true in that the withdrawal is something that is forced onto the elderly by society, then the well-adjusted old person is the one who maintains his activities.

This prediction form the disengagement theory that good adjustment and satisfaction in old age are characterized by withdrawal has not been confirmed and the results of investigations into this issue show a general trend in the reverse direction (Havighurst et al., 1968; Maddox and Eisdorfer, 1962). On the other hand, in further work leading from the disengagement theory the Chicago group (Neugarten et al., 1964, 1968) have come to the conclusion that high life satisfaction in old age is not invariably linked to the maintenance of involvement in outside activities and social links, but that individuals with differing basic temperaments find their maximal adjustment in old age in different ways.

SLOWNESS AND MOTOR PERFORMANCE

An obvious characteristic of the behaviour of the elderly and which affects many aspects of functioning is slowness. Slowness has already been encountered as a contributory factor in intellectual decline and other cognitive functions and it is at least as manifest in motor tasks. For example there have been a large number of studies like that of Botwinick *et al.* (1957) which have demonstrated that reaction time decreases throughout adult life.

An important question in relation to slowing on motor tasks, and which has often been reviewed (e.g., Welford, 1959 and 1962; Botwinick, 1973), is whether slowing is due to impaired sensory and effector processes or is due to a retardation in more-central decision processes which control movement. The evidence on this point is fairly clear with only very few exceptions (Waugh *et al.*, 1973). Experiments on reaction time by Botwinick (1971) and by Birren and Botwinick (1955), have showed that varying the intensity of the reaction time stimulus or the length of the motor pathway involved in the response have very little effect (except possibly at extreme values) in altering the relative deterioration in speed of reaction time found in elderly subjects. These results imply that slowing is a central rather than a peripheral phenomenon. Also, this conclusion is not limited to the type of experimental technique or type of response used by Botwinick and his colleagues because Singleton (1954) reached the same conclusion using a continuous motor task, rather than the simple, discrete reaction-time response, and a rather different method of estimating the contribution of central and peripheral components in the total response.

Having accepted that it is largely central processes that are responsible for the slowing of motor responses, is it possible to refine this any further? There is not a great deal of evidence but one factor that seems to be at least contributary is that of expectancy or 'set' (Botwinick, 1973). Botwinick and Thompson (1966) varied the preparatory interval between a warning stimulus and the reaction-time stimulus and found that it had an appreciable effect. This, and related work by Botwinick and his colleagues (see Botwinick, 1973) has confirmed that elderly subjects, especially men (the picture was a little different for women but this may well have been because of an experimental artifact), had particular difficulty with both long and short preparatory intervals as opposed to those of intermediate length. Botwinick (1973) has concluded that the elderly are less capable of maintaining set for long periods and also have more difficulty in learning how to 'get set' quickly.

THEORIES OF NORMAL AGEING

It would be wrong to leave our discussion of normal ageing without at least some mention of theories of ageing. The most actively developed and researched theories of normal ageing (see Busse, 1969; Comfort, 1973) are biological and have little direct implication for the psychological aspects of gerontology as yet. For completeness we need only mention that these biological theories involve such principles as the idea that in dividing cells, the new cells in old animals are not as efficient as the new cells in younger animals, or the notion that irreplaceable cells (e.g., neurones in the brain) are either lost or become less effective. The specific biological theories try to explain how these things might come to pass.

What is required for psychological studies of ageing are theories that explain the behavioural changes, or some aspects of them, in terms of a smaller number of key processes. This is, of course, assuming that the basic mechanisms underlying the ageing process are biological in nature. There are few psychological theories and some of those that do exist are too vague to be of much heuristic value, e.g. the hypothesis that the older person's brain has to work against a lower signal-to-noise ratio (Welford, 1962). Looking for a grand psychological theory of ageing that will encompass everything is likely to be fruitless but more specific theories dealing with certain aspects of behaviour are much more likely to be successful and can inspire further investigation. An example already encountered is the disengagement theory in the area of personality and social change. Another theoretical approach that could be worthwhile in the field of cognitive changes is Rabbitt's (1968) analogy between the ageing individual and an ageing computer in that both are slower to process information and do so with less efficiency. On the whole, theories have not had a large impact on the psychological aspects of gerontology.

GENERAL COMMENT ON NORMAL AGEING

This necessarily brief and selective review of behavioural changes associated with ageing has shown, if nothing else, how wide ranging these changes are. It would not be appropriate to try and summarize these changes but some general comments and qualifications are in order.

One question that has been raised in different ways at different times is whether the observed age changes are not just an epiphenomenon. In particular it has been suggested that older subjects are less likely to be well motivated to perform in tests and experiments and that this could account for the lowered levels of performance over a wide range of tasks.

Motivation is not the easiest of variables to deal with experimentally and so this idea is difficult to put to the test. There are two main lines of argument against the use of motivation as a complete explanation of all age-produced behaviour changes. The first is that lowered motivation might be expected to affect all tasks to a more or less equal degree (this is also assuming that we are not dealing with a situation in which the younger subject might be considered to be 'overmotivated' and where a reduction in motivation might be expected to enhance performance). Inglis et al. (1968) used this approach in claiming that the results of their dichotic listening experiments could not be explained in motivational terms because it was largely only the second set of stimuli to be reported which were affected by ageing. Of more direct relevance to the problem of motivation it would be expected that, in a signal detection analysis of age changes in memory, motivation would tend to affect the decision criteria used and not the level of discriminability of the stimuli. However this was not borne out by Gordon and Clark (1974) whose data suggested that their older group were definitely less able to detect previously learned information.

The second type of argument is based on the rationale that if older subjects perform badly because of poor motivation, then enhancing motivation should appreciably enhance their performance. Younger subjects must be presumed to be nearer their optimum level of motivation and therefore will not have as much room for improvement if their motivation is increased. There are at least two experiments in which performance on a particular task has been studied in both younger and older subjects under neutral conditions as well as under conditions of alleged heightened motivation. Ganzler (1964) looked at the time spent in completing questionnaires by patients in an American Veterans Administration hospital. Extra motivation was induced by giving subjects a strong reminder of the then commonly-expressed opinion in certain sections of the American press that the Veterans Administration institutions contained a lot of patients who were merely 'spongers on society'. They were then told that the only way that they could combat this erroneous impression was to cooperate with the hospital authorities in doing everything that they were asked to do as carefully and well as they could. In another study Botwinick *et al.* (1958) measured reaction times and provided extra motivation by applying a mild electric shock to the subject whenever his response time dropped below a certain level. In both these experiments the procedures designed to increase motivation had a beneficial effect on performance but the effect was equal for both old and young subjects.

The available evidence is therefore not in keeping with the hypothesis that poor motivation is the cause of the psychological changes associated with ageing. On the other hand, anyone who is particularly enamoured of this hypothesis could point to possible inadequacies in these experiments and also easily set forth further assumptions about the way in which motivation acts withoutout giving up the basic theory. It could also be argued that one of the most powerful arguments against motivation, or any other similar variable, as a major explanation of age changes is simply just this last point. To stretch the explanation to fit all the varied findings would entail too many improbable assumptions and may even end up by being a more complex explanation because of these than would any position which argued that ageing produces a range of deficits. Of course, this is not to claim that lowered motivation in the elderly cannot be partly responsible for any reductions in performance. It is just extremely unlikely that it is the major factor underlying most of the widely investigated phenomena.

A second type of underlying factor that is of great importance in ageing and which undoubtedly can affect psychological variables is that of health. It is extensively documented (e.g., Birren, 1964; Botwinick, 1973) that the health of older people is less good and the sensory systems in particular function less efficiently. These things cannot but place limits on the behavioural capacities of old people. Diseases of the cardiovascular system become increasingly common with age and have been established as producing psychological deficits (Abrahams and Birren, 1973; Wilkie and Eisdorfer, 1971).

This also has implications for what we understand as 'normal ageing'. Since sensory changes and certain disease processes are so common in the elderly it is difficult to decide what is a necessary part of the ageing process and what is the product of incidental features.

A final point concerns the nature of the data that have been presented. Apart from the field of intelligence, most comes from cross-sectional data and we have already seen the dangers of relying too heavily on this method. Also, as is the case with most areas of psychology, discussion is concerned almost exclusively with average data. The individual who fits the average picture is so rarely encountered that the 'average man' is sometimes regarded as a joke. This point is even more true in the case of ageing because on many measures, although not all, not only does the average level of performance decline but the range of variability increases. The average must then reflect a proportion who show much larger changes and a proportion who show very little change. This is also borne out by the fact that comparisons of old and young usually reveal large overlaps in the data.

Part Two
The Psychological Changes in Dementia

3
Intellectual Changes in Dementia

The very term 'dementia' implies above all else a deterioration in intellectual functioning. It is therefore to be expected that patients with dementia would show a lower level of performance on all types of intellectual task including the standardized tests of intelligence. In fact if no appreciable decline were observed we would be forced either to reconsider our concept of dementia or seriously to question the validity of the psychological tests.

Without being too arbitrary it is possible to classify research into the intellectual changes in dementia into two main categories. The first involves the straightforward application of various well-known standardized tests of intelligence to groups of dements and possibly also to control groups as well. The weakness of this approach is that, beyond confirming the obvious decline in IQ in dementia, it tells us little about the much more interesting question of the nature of the change in intellectual functioning. The second type of investigation, which may still employ one or more of the usual intelligence tests, is directed towards elucidating the nature of intellectual change. Here the emphasis is often on more fundamental features alleged to underlie intellectual activity.

Despite the central position that intellectual change must have within the study of dementia, it is a topic which has gone very much out of fashion and there is very little recent literature. For this reason much of the present chapter will carry a rather old fashioned air. The newer approaches to the study of intellectual change in normal ageing which were briefly outlined in the previous chapter have generally not been applied to the abnormalities of ageing. Possibly the clinical psychologist's quite-reasonable rejection of the role of administering intelligence and other tests has turned him away from other ways of looking at intellectual change.

THE PERFORMANCE OF DEMENTED PATIENTS ON STANDARDIZED TESTS OF INTELLIGENCE

Because intelligence tests have been administered frequently, if not always sensibly, in clinical practice the collation of test scores and IQs can present the easiest of all possible investigations for the psychologist. As a result there are a large number of cited figures and they do not warrant individual discussion. Those given in the tables and upon which the subsequent comments are based, probably represent the majority of published investigations which meet certain fairly minimal criteria concerning the descriptions of the subject

TABLE 3

Summary of studies applying the Wechsler intelligence scales to groups of
demented patients expressed as mean IQs

	N	Verbal	Performance	Full scale
Wechsler Bellevue				
Botwinnick and Birren (1951a)	31	—	—	84·1
Cleveland and Dysinger (1944)	17	89·5	52·8	—
Dorken and Greenbloom (1953)	67	—	—	77·6
Halstead (1943)	20	—	—	106
Lovett-Doust *et al.* (1953)	89	—	—	84·5
WAIS				
Bolton *et al.* (1966)	47	83·6	77·1	79·7
Kendrick *et al.* (1965)	20	93·1	79·2	—
Kendrick and Post (1967)	10	96·0	79·5	—
Miller (unpublished)	20	78·1	68·8	72·5
Sanderson and Inglis (1961)	15	89·0	—	—

populations used, the measures administered, and the results obtained. In
view of the consistency of the picture obtained the results of any overlooked
reports are not likely to affect the conclusions drawn.

The results of several investigations in which the Wechsler intelligence
scales (either the Wechsler–Bellevue or the later Wechsler Adult Intelligence
Scale) have been applied to demented subjects are shown in Table 3. It can
readily be seen that, with the exception of Halstead (1943), all report average
IQs below the expected mean for the population of 100. Where control groups
have also been tested, the dements invariably emerge with lower scores. As
mentioned above these findings are hardly surprising.

The mean full scale IQ of 106 on the Wechsler–Bellevue scale found by
Halstead (1943) requires some explanation. In the first place Halstead based
his estimate of IQ on only three out of the complete set of ten subtests. This
would greatly increase the error of measurement. Secondly, since Halstead
used no control group, the assumption is being made, as in the other studies
which use no control group, that the sample is drawn from a population that
would have had the usual overall population mean IQ of 100 but for the onset of
their illness. In any individual case this assumption is probably only approximately true and it could well be that Halstead's particular sample happened
to be drawn from subjects of generally about average premorbid intellectual
levels. Slightly against this is the information which Halstead gives about the
socioeconomic background of his sample, showing that this was probably not
markedly different from the normal population in having a predominance of
unskilled workers and only one subject with a professional background. What
ever the reason for this one atypical result, which is quite possibly an artifact,
it is of little significance when viewed against other results.

These low IQ levels only confirm the obvious prediction about dementia and
the interesting point is what information can be derived from them about the

nature of intellectual decline in dementia. One indication from Table 3 is that where it is possible to compare Wechsler verbal and performance IQs, the performance IQs are always lower. There are a number of possible reasons for this discrepancy. The first is that speed is generally an important factor in the subtests comprising the performance scale. Within the limits of the test administrator's patience and the subjects' persistence speed is of very little significance for most of the verbal subtests. Thus the demented subject may be particularly impaired on speeded tests. One point against regarding slowing of cognitive functions as being of critical importance in this issue comes from the reports of data from the Mill Hill Vocabulary Scale and Progressive Matrices. These will be considered below but the key point for the present is that neither of these tests are speeded but dements still show a similar tendency towards higher scores on the more verbal of these two tests. The writer's impression, gained from testing a large number of demented patients, is that speed is not the crucial factor in poor performance scores. If it were, demented subjects would be expected to achieve correct solutions to the various problems but fail to get there within the time limit. When they fail they tend to fail completely, giving the impression that more generous time limits would not result in a correct solution.

There are two other possible explanations of the verbal-performance discrepancy. The performance scale uses subtests involving the manipulation of visuospatial relationships and these may be especially impaired in dementia. The final explanation lies in the fact that the items in the verbal scale tend to relate to well practised verbal and arithmetical activities and overlearned pieces of information. In contrast, the performance scale items are much less familiar and require the subject to adjust to new situations. Although demented subjects are impaired in the handling of spatial relationships (see Chapter 5), the latter explanation in terms of an inability to learn to cope with new types of situation is particularly plausible in the light of the marked disturbances in acquisition that have been demonstrated in dementia.

Further analysis of data from the Wechsler intelligence scales can be carried out by looking at scores on the 10 or 11 individual subtests that make up the full scale. Analysis of subtest scores has enjoyed a certain popularity with these psychologists interested in all types of psychopathology but it suffers from two

TABLE 4

Mean WAIS age corrected subtest scores with their standard deviations from a series of 20 cases of presenile dementia (author's previously unpublished data)

	Mean	S.D.		Mean	S.D.
Information	6·40	2·66	Digit Symbol	3·35	3·90
Comprehension	5·80	4·09	Picture Completion	6·35	3·33
Arithmetic	5·95	2·80	Block Design	4·25	3·67
Similarities	5·35	4·07	Picture Arrangement	3·10	3·48
Digit Span	6·25	3·48	Object Assembly	3·50	3·12
Vocabulary	8·00	3·21			

major drawbacks: firstly there is little reliable information on the specific abilities being tapped by the various subtests, and secondly subtest scores are rather unreliable. This makes for a wide range of variation in subtest data. One example of subtest scores will suffice. Table 4 shows the mean, age-corrected, subtest scores of a previously unpublished series of 20 cases of presenile dementia tested on the Wechsler Adult Intelligence Scale by the present author. (The expected mean subtest score for the normal population is 10·0 with a standard deviation of 3·0.)

Limited conclusions can be drawn from this data other than the obvious fact that all the values are below the expected mean of 10·0. Despite the mean scores being compressed into the lower half of the scale, all but two of the subtests have standard deviations above the normal value of 3·0. Usually compression of scores in this way would be expected to decrease the amount of variation. This shows the very high variability between individual patients with dementia and rules out the notion that there might be a characteristic profile of subtest scores which is shown by most patients with dementia.

The idea that vocabulary scores might be an indicator of premorbid intelligence has an important place in the psychological assessment of dementia and will be examined in Chapter 8. For the present it is worth noting that whilst the vocabulary subtest has, on average, the highest score there is still some decline in vocabulary. With the exception of Picture Completion the subtests with the lowest scores all belong to the performance scale. These specific subtests appear to have no obvious feature in common other than those already mentioned as possible explanations of the verbal-performance discrepancy.

A further set of tests that have been used extensively on groups of demented subjects are the Mill Hill Vocabulary Scale and the Progressive Materices test. A number of sets of published data are summarized in Table 5 but again, this is not claimed to be an exhaustive list. The conclusions that can be drawn from this table echo those resulting from the examination of reports of the use of the Wechsler scales.

TABLE 5

Summary of studies applying the Mill Hill Vocabulary Scale and Progressive Matrices expressed as mean scores (direction of relationship takes normative data into account)

	N	Mill Hill	Progressive Matrices	Relationship
Hopkins and Roth (1953)	14	—	4·8	—
Kendrick et al. (1967)	20	100·6[a]	—	MH > PM
Kendrick and Post (1965)	10	—	86·33[a]	MH > PM
Newcombe and Steinberg (1964)	9	21·1[b]	21·4	MH > PM
Orme (1957)	25	41·64	15·0	MH > PM
Roth and Hopkins (1953)	12	—	4·5	—

[a]Score converted to IQ equivalent (original paper does not give raw scores).
[b]Score based on half test only.

The mean scores cited are generally below those expected on the basis of the general population and this is especially true of scores on the Progressive Matrices test (where raw scores are cited conclusions are based on reference to published norms). Where control groups were tested, the demented group invariably had lower scores and there is a marked tendency for a discrepancy between Mill Hill and Matrices scores in favour of the former. Similar reasons to those suggested for the Wechsler verbal-performance discrepancy can be advanced to explain this, with the exception of speed which is not an important factor in either of these two tests. At face value the Matrices is certainly the less verbal and more spatially oriented test and it seems to present the subject with a rather more novel situation.

Further investigations which merely apply intelligence tests to a population of subjects with dementia and then compare the results with control groups are not likely to achieve anything more. There is one possible exception to this statement and that is the long-term prospective study which picks up a sample of early cases and re-tests them at suitable intervals. This would then allow the pattern of change in test scores to be looked at as the disease progresses. Such information would be useful in trying to determine whether dementia was merely an accelerated ageing of the nervous system (see Chapter 7). There is only one report of the repeated administration of intelligence tests (Kendrick and Post, 1967) but this investigation was not designed with the present purpose in mind and so the test–re-test intervals were too short to be of value in this context.

ATTEMPTS TO DESCRIBE THE NATURE OF THE INTELLECTUAL CHANGE IN DEMENTIA

An extension of the pure psychometric approach, dealt with above, is the attempt to apply techniques which will give some hint as to the underlying nature or central feature of intellectual change in dementia. The earliest research of this type involved assumptions about the occurrence of dementia that could not be accepted today. The best illustration of this comes from the term 'dementia praecox' which was used to label what we would now describe as schizophrenia. It contains the explicit assumption that patients with this particular functional psychosis are dementing in the same sort of way as are those with the organic dementias.

Given this assumption, current at the time at which they were writing, it is not surprising that Hart and Spearman (1914) used a wide range of subjects with both functional and organic psychoses as though they were a fairly homogeneous population. Their paper is therefore mainly of historical interest as being the first published experimental attempt to define the nature of dementia more clearly.

Hart and Spearman applied a wide range of mental tests to a selection of abnormal subjects and a group of normal individuals. The variation in test performance within the abnormal group was found to be no greater than that shown by the controls. This is surprising in view of the very varied sample of subjects in the abnormal group and the common later finding that abnormal groups tend to give a greater degree of variation on many measures (see Payne, 1960). Using Spearman's theory of intellectual functioning which postulates a general intellectual factor and a number of subordinate factors, they argued that the findings were consistent with the notion that dementia represents a decline in the general factor. However, these authors did allow that different psychiatric conditions might also produce deficits in particular specific factors.

At first sight Brody (1942) appears to have been using a concept of dementia that is akin to the present one although his actual selection of subjects gives cause for concern. This paper, which purports to be a study of dementia, contains a table showing the diagnosis of his 50–69-year-old hospitalized subjects *before* they started dementing. Most of these diagnoses consist of functional psychiatric disorders. This makes the reader wonder whether, in some cases at least, Brody was confusing dementia with the intellectual deterioration which may occur as a consequence of long-standing functional psychosis or its resultant institutionalization. Brody administered a varied battery of tests to his subjects which included a vocabulary test, the Standford–Binet Intelligence Scale Form L, and other verbal and non-verbal tests. Vocabulary was found to be well maintained in dementia but, apart from this, no specific pattern of change in test scores was noted. Brody also commented in detail upon the qualitative features of his subjects' performance on these tests. He claimed, amongst other things, that dementia produced slowness, thinking that was less abstract, and a reduction of insight into the nature of the tests.

The remaining published reports raise a number of issues most of which have yet to be convincingly resolved. The first of these is whether the intellectual performance of demented subjects is qualitatively different from that of the normal person. It is of some significance in indicating the hazards of research in this area that one author, Margaret Davies Eysenck, was able to publish results coming down on both sides of this question within the same year.

Eysenck (1945a) gave Raven's Progressive Matrices test to a large number of patients with senile dementia and compared their performance with normal controls and also with children. All three types of subject showed a similar order of difficulty in the test items. The author also looked at the pattern of errors produced by the different types of subject. This is easy to do with the Progressive Matrices because each item presents the subject with a set of alternatives from which the correct one is to be chosen. Again there was no indication that where errors were made the demented subject was likely to choose a different incorrect alternative from the other types of subject. It must be concluded that this investigation gives no indication of a different pattern of intellectual performance in dementia. On the other hand the use of a single test which utilizes a homogeneous set of items throughout gives little scope for differences of this sort to be shown up.

In her other investigation (Eysenck, 1945b) a large battery of tests was administered to 75 patients with senile dementia who may well have been an overlapping group with that used in the investigation described immediately above. The battery included tests of intelligence, memory, general knowledge, and motor performance. A form of factor analysis was carried out on the data. This revealed a general factor which accounted for a large proportion of the variance and three specific factors. The finding of a general factor is consistent with results obtained from similar analyses using normal subjects but its nature was rather different. Using Cattell's (1943) distinction between fluid and crystallized ability, it appeared to Eysenck that the general factor in dements was much more highly saturated with tests of crystallized ability.

Eysenck's (1945b) paper gives at least a hint that intellectual structure may show qualitative changes in dementia. Another approach to this issue is to analyse patterns of subtest scores derived from the Wechsler intelligence scales to see if these differ from those to be expected as a result of normal ageing. Botwinick and Birren (1951b), and Dorken and Greenbloom (1953) agree in finding differences whilst Rabin (1945) and Whitehead (1973b) did not. Whether there really are qualitative differences between the changes found in dementia and those of normal ageing will be taken up in greater detail in Chapter Seven.

A related issue is the comparison of the changes observed in dementia with occurring in other psychiatric abnormalities. Direct evidence on this point is sparse although the findings in dementia do generally differ from those associated with studies of other organic and functional psychiatric disorders (e.g., Payne, 1973). Cameron (1938) did describe differences between patients with senile dementia and patients with other types of psychiatric disorder. He required his subjects to complete sentences whose opening words were provided (e.g., 'A man fell down in the road because . . . . '). It seemed that as a general rule the responses of demented subjects showed a remarkable preservation of social functioning despite their memory disturbances and disorientation. The main abnormality described was a tendency to evade the point which Cameron interpreted as a possible defence against their inadequacies. Using an analysis of subtest scores on the Wechsler Adult Intelligence Scale, Aminoff et al. (1975) concluded that there were differences in intellectual performance between patients with Huntington's chorea and other presenile dementias.

Assuming that impairments may occur which are qualitatively different from the changes found in normal ageing and which are specific to dementia (i.e., which cannot be attributed to any general 'illness' factor) other problems arise. Can the change in dementia be described as an alteration in a single variable or is the intellectual change much more complex than this? How can this change best be described?

One paper which appears to give direct evidence as to the number of dimensions involved in intellectual change is that of Dixon (1965). Dixon factor analysed data from a larger number of brief tests given to 70 elderly subjects with varying degrees of dementia. A single factor was found to account for a very high proportion of the total variance and Dixon concludes that intellectual deterioration must therefore occur along a single dimension.

Dixon's use of brief tests means that these were probably of low reliability and hence there would be a high proportion of the total variance in the data that could be attributed to error. This would bias the analysis towards giving the observed result. In addition, factor analytic studies of this type are always open to criticism with regard to the representativeness of the measures used and the extent to which the data fit the statistical assumptions involved. A different battery of tests applied to a different sample might well give a different result judging by factor analytic investigations in other areas and for this reason Dixon's report cannot be taken as definitive.

A paper of not quite such direct interest with regard to the issue under discussion is that of Gustafson and Hagberg (1975). These authors factor analysed the data obtained from applying various psychiatric, psychological and neurological examinations to 57 cases of presenile dementia. In all, 67 variables were used in the analysis which yielded no less than 14 factors. Of these, at least three appeared to have a definite intellectual component and these were labelled 'amnesia–apraxia', 'amnesia–confusion', and 'agraphia–alexia'. At first sight this definitely contradicts Dixon's conclusion that intellectual change in dementia involves only a single dimension, but it must also be acknowledged that the inclusion of non-psychological variables in the analysis probably distorted the picture.

Regardless of whether intellectual decline occurs along one or more dimensions we are still faced with the difficulty of deciding just what these dimensions are. There is no current information on this point and those who have attempted to tackle this issue in the past have naturally used concepts appropriate to the time at which their investigations were carried out. One distinction that has been used is that between 'fluid' and 'crystallized' intelligence in Cattell's (1943) terminology. We have already seen that Eysenck (1945b) has suggested that demented subjects might be particularly impaired in fluid intelligence.

Although not himself utilizing Cattell's terminology, Halstead (1943) provides evidence which he interprets in a similar way and which is consistent with Eysenck (1945b). Halstead had 20 'less seriously demented' elderly patients to whom he administered a number of tests. He found that the tests showing the greatest impairment were those in which the subject could not use old mental habits and had to adapt to unfamiliar situations or ways of thinking. Unfortunately the effective comparison was between his experimental group and the average performance of younger normal subjects and this confounds the effects of ageing with those of dementia.

Another possible way of categorizing the intellectual performance of demented patients is by using Goldstein's concept of concrete as opposed to abstract thinking, and as tested for by the use of Goldstein and Scheerer's (1941) object sorting tests. The first investigators to apply these tests to demented subjects were Cleveland and Dysinger (1944). They found that demented subjects had a strong tendency to group the objects concretely and not on a conceptual basis (e.g., by shape or material out of which they were constructed.) A few could sort abstractly if the choice was narrowed to a state in which only a single conceptual principle was possible. The subjects were also given the Wechsler–Bellevue Intelligence Scale, and Cleveland and Dysigner emphasize that some of their sample could supply abstract principles in answer to questions from the similarities subtest. Even these were unable to put their capacity to use abstract principles into effect when carrying out the sorting tests.

Although not using the Goldstein–Scheerer sorting tests, Pinkerton and Kelly (1952) invoke the notion of a loss of abstract ability in a qualitative analysis of the response produced by demented subjects on the Progressive Matrices test. Further qualified support comes from Hopkins and Post (1955) who applied the Goldstein–Scheerer sorting tests to elderly psychiatric patients with functional psychiatric disorders. However, in their discussion of the results they do refer to previous work in which the tests were also applied to demented subjects. Apparently the previous demented sample had turned out to be extremely concrete according to Goldstein and Scheerer's (1941) criteria. The main body of Hopkins and Post's paper reveals that very few of their elderly subjects with functional psychiatric disorders or even elderly normals were able to produce consistently abstract sorting. Thus it may be that concrete thinking is not the sole prerogative of demented subjects in elderly populations and the demented subject may only differ in degree from his normal counterpart as far as this variable is concerned.

COMMENT

Although a decline in intellectual powers is central to the concept of dementia it has not attracted a great deal of psychological research. The straightforward examination of the IQ levels of demented subjects very readily confirms that the expected intellectual deterioration does exist and this easy demonstration may possibly have satisfied many who might otherwise have been more curious. The real challenge of the intellectual decline in dementia (as of the disturbance in many other functions) is not in proving that change has occurred but in specifying the underlying nature of that change in greater detail.

With regard to this wider question there is no firm evidence and only a number of suggestions derived from rather old fashioned research. Many writers who have tackled the issue argue that the nature of intellectual performance in dementia is qualitatively different from that of normal subjects of a similar age. This point will be taken up in a much wider context in Chapter 7, but for the present we may assume that this viewpoint is more likely to be true than its corresponding null hypothesis. The verbal-performance discrepancy on the Wechsler intelligence scales is a consistent finding which gives some possible leads to the nature of any difference in intellectual structure but there is a dearth of work following this up. The notions of concrete thinking and crystallized ability have also been invoked but many of the studies are not very convincing and neither has gained a definite acceptance in this context.

The work described in this chapter has been limited to investigations using the conventional types of psychometric test which purport to measure intellectual functioning. This limitation may partly account for the disappointing lack of firm conclusions and for the dearth of interest in these problems in recent years. The psychometric approach is restricted by the availability of suitable, valid tests. Whilst such instruments can be found to measure general factors of intelligence they are very much less readily available when more specific intellectual skills are to be examined. This is especially so where the subject population is elderly. The alternative approach is to study the thought processes of demented subjects by means of the experimental techniques commonly used by experimental psychologists to investigate normal cognitive functioning. In particular the newer ways of approaching the issue of normal intellectual changes with ageing, which were briefly referred to in Chapter 2, have not been applied to abnormal ageing.

A final point is that any subdivision of psychological processes is inevitably arbitrary. Intellectual functioning does not conveniently separate itself from more specific topics such as the understanding of spatial relationships and language which are covered in Chapter 5. Before going on to these we will examine the other outstanding psychological change in dementia which is that occurring in memory.

4
Memory

General intellectual deterioration must be considered the *sine qua non* of dementia but also extremely important is the memory disturbance which is not infrequently the first manifestation of a dementing illness. In discussing the psychopathology of dementia, Zangwill (1964) claims that not all demented patients show memory defects as assessed by psychometric tests. Such a belief is only tenable if applied to the earliest stages of dementia and even then it is rather dubious. Whilst it is impossible finally to disprove Zangwill's theory by showing that every case does involve some memory impairment, the evidence to be described in this chapter points so overwhelmingly to a marked decline in memory as a result of dementia that the universality of this type of disturbance seems a much more reasonable assumption.

The tradition in experimental psychology has been to separate the study of verbal memory from the study of the learning and retention of non-verbal activities such as motor skills and work following the operant and classical conditioning paradigms. Not unnaturally, psychologists interested in abnormal behaviour have tended to keep the same distinctions as those used by their colleagues in general experimental psychology. As far as dementia is concerned there has been an appreciable amount of work following the verbal learning/memory tradition and this approach will be dealt with in this chapter. The rather smaller output related to other aspects of learning and memory will be covered in Chapter 5.

As was the case with intellectual deterioration in the previous chapter, the important issue is not demonstrating that memory losses occur in dementia but in elucidating their nature. In attempting to do this, problems arise over and above those inherent in the task itself. There have been few systematic series of investigations into memory changes in dementia. This means that often isolated experiments using a variety of techniques have to be reconciled with one another. The only systematic studies are those of Inglis and his associates and those of the present author. These two sets of experiments will therefore be considered separately after the discussion of the other evidence. Another problem which requires special comment is that of models of memory.

MODELS OF MEMORY

Dealing with experimental work on abnormalities of memory requires a model of normal memory. To argue an effective case for the use of any particular model of normal memory upon which to base subsequent discussion would involve a digression of such proportions as to swamp the rest of this chapter. The model assumed here is, in general terms, one that is described and used by many experimental psychologists working in the field of normal memory (e.g., Broadbent, 1970). It involves the division of memory into a temporary short-term store of limited capacity and a more permanent, long-term, store. The question of an iconic memory preceding the short-term store as indicated by the experiments of Sperling (1960), Averbach and Coriell (1961), and subsequent work in that tradition (for a recent review see Coltheart, 1972), does not really arise in the present context since no work dealing with iconic memory in abnormal subjects has yet been reported.

The distinction between short-term and long-term memory is favoured here for a number of reasons. Prominent amongst these is the fact that many of the experimental studies of memory in dementia have assumed this distinction. Those like Gruneberg (1970), who favour a unitary theory of memory storage, can reinterpret the information presented without too much difficulty according to their own assumptions about the nature of memory.

CLINICAL EVALUATIONS OF THE MEMORY DISORDER IN DEMENTIA

Standard textbooks of psychiatry, neurology, and geriatrics often give clinical descriptions of the memory disorder in dementia. These descriptions will not be regurgitated here and a summary has already been provided in Chapter One. A small number of clinicians have attempted to go beyond mere description and to try to analyse the nature of the memory disorder based on clinical evidence. Whilst such analyses cannot be regarded as yielding firm conclusions, and can rightly be criticized for lack of objectivity, clinical insights are not necessarily wrong and can be a useful source of hypotheses for experimental evaluation (McGhie, 1973).

Boyd (1936) reported an extensive clinical examination of psychological factors in a 54-year-old male subject with Alzheimer's disease. He concluded that it was memory for recent events that was affected and that remote memory remained intact. This is a not uncommon impression, but Boyd was also impressed by the marked degree of the memory impairment as compared with the apparently milder decline in general intellectual functioning.

Kral (1958, 1962 and 1966) has argued on both clinical and experimental grounds that two types of memory disturbance can be found in old age. These he refers to as 'benign' and 'malignant'. The benign memory impairment is, as its name implies, relatively mild and consists of the occasional inability to recall certain details of information. These details usually belong to the remote rather than the recent past and are lost to the subject only on particular occasions. The subject is aware of his inability to recall and may apologize or use circumlocutions to get round the problem. The same detail is often recalled with normal facility on a later occasion. Kral cites as an example of benign memory impairment an old lady who described going to her son's wedding some years previously but who could not recall the name of the city in which the wedding had taken place. On being examined later she had no difficulty at all in providing the name of the city.

In contrast malignant memory impairment is more marked for items from the recent past and whole sequences are lost rather than just details as in benign memory impairment. The malignant form also leads to disorientation and eventually to a loss of remote events although items of information with strong emotional connotations may be relatively well preserved. Kral draws parallels between this form of memory impairment and the dysmnesic syndrome and even goes as far as to use the term 'senile Korsakoff'.

These two forms of memory impairment are distinguished in a number of other ways. The sexes are equally represented in the benign type whilst females predominate in the malignant. The malignant type is also associated with a reduced life expectancy. With regard to the specific nature of the memory impairment Kral argues that the benign type is due to difficulties in recall. The malignant form is more complex. Kral suggests that recall is probably no more affected than in the benign type but the registration of information is also considered to be reduced in efficiency. Assuming that his descriptions have some validity, the predominantly clinical data used by Kral do not convincingly demonstrate that he is dealing with two distinct types of memory disorder rather than merely describing the milder and more advanced forms of the same process. The exact relationship between the benign type of memory disorder and the normal decline in memory due to age is not spelled out.

EARLY EXPERIMENTAL STUDIES

These are distinguished from later investigations by their methodology and by the general concept of memory that appears to underly the experiments. The later experimental work is largely within the framework of the general model of memory described above. Not surprisingly, later investigators use techniques currently in use within the mainstream of experimental psychology. These things are not the case in the earlier experiments.

Possibly the earliest experimental study of memory in dementia is that of Moore (1919). He used sets of eight stimuli (objects, pictures of objects, and printed and spoken words) presented at a rate of one every 2 seconds. The subjects were predominantly cases of senile dementia but the group did contain some patients with other diagnoses. Following the presentation of a set of stimuli the subjects were asked for an immediate recall of what they had seen or heard. After a one-minute interval filled by mental arithmetic, a delayed recall was also requested to assess 'retention'. A test of 'perception' was also administered and this involved noting the time taken to 'recognize' (i.e., name) pictures of objects. (Although claimed to be a test of perception, this last task could obviously be affected by a number of variables other than perception, e.g. a dysphasic type of impairment in supplying names.) Moore concluded that immediate memory, retention, and perception (as defined by his experimental technique) tend to deteriorate together. This tendency is not universal according to Moore because some subjects deteriorate more in one aspect than in the others. Moore also stressed that his tests of immediate memory and retention were not measuring the same thing. Unfortunately this conclusion, like all his others, has to be considered in the light of techniques that are inadequate by present day standards and the fact that no control subjects were used.

A rather more detailed investigation was reported not very long after Moore by Liljencrantz (1922). Liljencrantz was concerned with trying to decide whether 'amnesia was due to faulty apprehension, faulty retention, or both'. This is a question that still excercises research workers in the field of amnesia and Liljencrantz based his attempt to find an answer on a wide range of subjects with memory impairments due to organic disease. Nevertheless a considerable proportion were patients with dementia. The experimental technique used pairs of pictures which depicted objects, persons or abstract designs. The pairs were pictorially similar without being identical. One of each pair was shown to the subject who then had to describe what he had seen (recall testing) or select the seen items from an array containing both the original stimuli and their paired pictures (recognition testing). Deficits were found with both forms of testing which Liljencrantz interpreted as showing that all organic amnesias are due to both faulty apprehension and faulty retention. Again the experimental techniques are not adequate for the intended purpose and all that can be reasonably concluded is that demented subjects fall down on both recognition and recall testing.

Following these two early experiments it might be expected that there would be an increasing flow of published reports of more and more sophisticated investigations in this field. Unfortunately this is not so and there is very little of note between Liljencrantz and the modern work to be considered in the following sections of this chapter.

Amongst the sparse offerings available in this period is a paper by Shakow et al. (1941). Although the statistical analyses for a sure interpretation are lacking, this report appears to indicate that memories relating to the distant past are as equally vulnerable to the effects of dementia as those of more recently experienced events. Testing for the retention of information from the distant past presents many methodological problems. Shakow et al. used such things as 'school information' which could well be more related to intelligence levels than memory per se. The lower vocabulary scores in the demented group as opposed to the normal controls could be taken to reflect the dements lower level of general intellectual functioning, and so explain their poor showing in the recall of distant items of information. Despite these criticisms the paper is of some interest as being the only occasion on which the clinical impression of dements having a relatively intact memory for distant events has been challenged. Since rather better techniques for assessing memory of the distant past have now been developed (Sanders and Warrington, 1971) a fresh attempt to replicate the findings of Shakow et al. would be of considerable interest.

The remaining publications require only passing mention. The very confused paper of Kral and Durost (1953) gives the impression of an investigation with no proper experimental design. Its only point of interest is that the authors claim a distinction whose basis they leave obscure between the type of memory disorder manifest in dementia and that shown by other conditions including Korsakoff's psychosis. Cameron (1940) also produces some evidence that the tendency of subjects to elaborate and distort remembered information, described by Bartlett (1932) in his classic study of normal memory, is speeded up and exaggerated in dementia.

THE WORK OF INGLIS AND HIS ASSOCIATES

In the work to be described here Inglis has been concerned to arrive at a better description or analysis of the memory defect in elderly patients with memory disorder. Inglis's preference for defining his subject populations in terms of their functional disturbances has already been discussed in Chapter 1. The point has been made that it is reasonable to regard his elderly patients with memory disorder as dements. In any case the proportion of senile patients with marked memory disturbances due to other causes and encountered in psychiatric practice is very small.

Inglis (1957) started by using paired-associate learning of the conventional type familiar to experimental psychologists. Here the subject has to learn to associate pairs of stimuli which may have no very obvious connection. If the stimuli used are words, the subject may have to respond 'pen' when the experimenter supplies the word 'cabbage'. Inglis used several tests of this type, all containing three pairs of words, but the sensory modality of presentation and method for testing of acquisition were varied. The stimuli were presented either auditorily or visually. When the first stimulus of a pair was given, the subject was either required to recall the word paired with it or to recognize this word from a set of alternatives. The experimental group took more trials to learn to criterion on all versions of the paired-associate test. The recall and recognition forms of the test both showed similar degrees of impairment in comparison with the normal control group. Not unreasonably, given the general state of knowledge at the time, this suggested to Inglis that the main deficit in his 'memory disordered' subjects lay in the acquisition of new information rather than its storage or recall. The main reason for this conclusion is that these latter aspects of memory might be expected to be differentially affected by the use of recall or recognition testing.

Inglis (1959a) attempted to confirm this finding of impaired acquisition and in addition to see if retention might also be impaired. The previously used technique of paired-associate learning was retained but this time only using an auditory presentation with recall of the paired word. In order to examine retention, the test was given twice since an improvement in learning on the second occasion could be used to indicate the amount of retention of the first learning trials. The initial difficulty in acquisition was again confirmed by the re-learning of the list which also indicated very little, if any, retention of what had been learned initially in the 'memory disordered' group. Other work with this paired associate form of testing was more directed at its diagnostic and prognostic significance and is therefore more appropriately dealt with elsewhere (see Chapters Six and Eight).

Feeling the need to specify the memory disorder more clearly, Inglis then went on to carry out further experiments using Broadbent's (1954) 'dichotic listening' technique. The essence of this technique is to present two separate messages simultaneously to the subject. The two messages are recorded on the separate channels of a twin-channel tape recorder and played through earphones such that the subject hears one message in one ear and the other message in the other ear. The 'messages' in these experiments were always lists of digits (with up to four digits per list) presented at a rate of two digits per second. The two messages, which are both of the same length and have no digits in common, are carefully synchronized. The first digit heard in one ear coincides exactly with the first digit heard in the other ear and so on for all the digits in the pair of messages.

The most common finding in dichotic listening experiments with young normal subjects is that when asked to recall everything that he has heard, the subject will repeat back one message before the other. He therefore seems to handle the two messages separately and not get the digits from the two messages mixed up. As might be expected the list (or ear) reported first contains far fewer errors. Broadbent (1958) explained these findings in terms of two hypothetical systems. The first, or 'p-system', is only able to pass information successively straight through the system. The second, 's-system' is a short-term memory store which can hold excess information when the 'p-system' is fully stretched. In the dichotic listening situation the first set of digits to be reported is processed immediately by the p-system. The set from the other ear is held temporarily in the storage provided by the s-system until the p-system has cleared the other set of digits.

Inglis (1960) hypothesized that a breakdown in Broadbent's s-system might lie behind the memory disorder in dementia. This is consistent with Inglis' previous work implicating the process of acquiring new information if it is further assumed that new information must pass through the s-system before reaching long-term storage.

Applying the dichotic listening technique to groups of elderly subjects both with and without memory disorder has produced substantially the same findings in each of a series of experiments (Caird and Hannah, 1964; Caird and Inglis, 1961; Inglis and Sanderson, 1961). Data from the first two of these experiments are summarized in the graphs shown in Figure 2. The results of the third experiment (Caird and Hannah, 1964) merely confirm the basic findings and this experiment will therefore not be specifically presented. It can be seen from Figure 2 that with lists up to three digits in length, there is little difference between the memory-disordered and control subjects in the ability to report the list recalled first. However, a difference in the list reported first

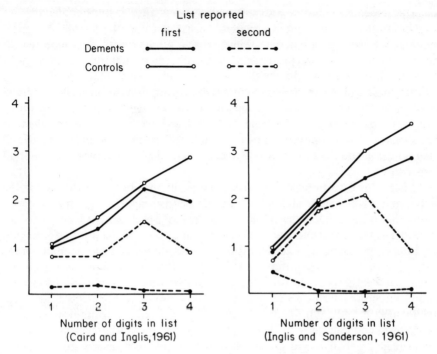

Figure 2. Report of digits in two dichotic listening experiments

does start to appear with four-digit lists. Just why this should be so is not explained by the authors.

It can also be seen from Figure 2 that Inglis' main hypothesis is supported in that memory-disordered subjects do recall the list reported second much less effectively. Given the theoretical assumptions under which these experiments were carried out, these results do support Inglis' notion of a short-term memory impairment.

The results of these experiments are reasonably clear cut as originally presented and as summarized by Inglis (1965, 1970). The basic problem is that the interpretation of dichotic listening phenomena used by Inglis and derived from Broadbent (1958) has been subject to serious challenge. A summary of some of the relevant arguments can be found in Broadbent (1971) but the important issue in the present context is that the interpretation of dichotic listening experiments with demented patients is left in the air.

THE PRESENT WRITER'S RESEARCH ON MEMORY IN DEMENTIA

An important preliminary point concerning Miller's investigations is that he has consistently used a somewhat different subject population to that used by most other workers in the field of dementia. Most other work is based on elderly demented subjects who are usually seen after institutionalization in psychiatric hospitals. Miller's samples consist of cases of presenile dementia undergoing investigation in neurological units. Whilst there is no sound reason to suppose that senile and presenile dements differ in the nature of their memory disorder, it is very likely that Miller's subjects were seen at a much earlier stage of the illness and usually before permanent institutionalization was considered necessary. The use of early cases has the disadvantage that any changes may not be so obvious and easy to demonstrate but there is the major advantage that the situation is not complicated by the grosser effects of generalized intellectual deterioration and the subject is able to cooperate in more complex experimental procedures.

Miller's investigations started from the point that both the then-available experimental evidence and clinical impressions implied that the memory deficit lay principally at the stage of acquisition. Specifically it was first of all considered that the demented subject was failing to establish new information in long-term memory. Consideration of the previous experimental work, including that of Inglis' group, revealed that an impaired short-term memory need not be the only reason why new information was not established in long-term storage. Not only could the short-term store be affected but there could also be an additional difficulty in transferring information between short-term and long-term memory. Concentration on this latter possibility was reinforced by then recently published reports of experiments involving the Montreal patient HM (e.g., Milner, *et al.*, 1968; Wickelgren, 1968) who had undergone bilateral mesial temporal lobe excisions for the relief of temporal lobe epilepsy. This operation resulted in an extremely severe amnesia. One suggestion about HM had been that short-term memory was intact but that he was incapable of getting new information into long-term memory (Miller, 1972a).

The first two experiments (Miller, 1971) were based on the free recall technique whereby the subject listens to a list of words and tries to recall as many of the words as he can, in any order, immediately following the presentation of the last word in the list. In this instance lists of twelve common, monosyllabic words were used and each list was initially presented at a rate of one word every $1\frac{1}{2}$ seconds. Plotting the probability of recall of a word against its position in the list gives a U-shaped curve. This is a well established phenomenon in normal subjects and is illustrated by the curve given by the control group in Figure 3. Glanzer and Cunitz (1966) have argued that the relatively good recall of the first few words in a list is due to these having passed through the short-term and into the long-term store. Their recall at the end of the list is assured because they have reached more permanent storage systems. Since new words arrive at the short-term store faster than they can be passed through to the long term store, the short-term store rapidly becomes overloaded, and many of the words in the middle portions of the list are lost. When the end of the list is reached, the last few words are still in short-term storage and can be readily retrieved. This then accounts for the elevation of the curve at the end of the list.

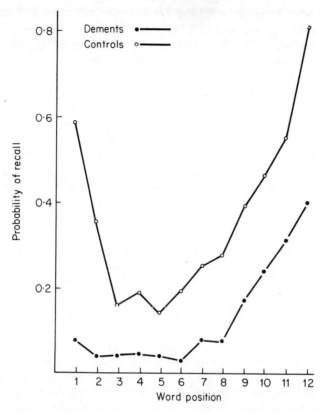

Figure 3. Recall of words as a function of their position in the
list. From Miller *Neuropsychologia*, **9**, 75 (1971) by permission
of Pergamon Press

In the first experiment described by Miller (1971), groups of patients with presenile dementia and normal control subjects each heard 20 lists and the graph showing probability of recall of the words against their position in the list is given by Figure 3. Using Glanzer and Cunitz's (1966) interpretation it can be seen that the control group has substantial elevations of the curve both at the beginning and at the end of the list. These reflect material that has been retrieved from the long-term store (the elevation at the beginning) and from the short-term store (elevation at the end). In contrast, the experimental group has a slightly depressed curve representing short-term store output which suggests a reduced capacity for the short-term store. Of greater interest is the almost total lack of an elevation of the curve at the beginning of the list which could be interpreted as showing that very little material is reaching the long-term store.

It is still not clear from this experiment whether the apparently much reduced ability of the demented subject to establish new material in the long-term store is due solely to a reduced capacity of the short-term store, or to an additional difficulty in transferring information between the two storage systems. This latter possibility was explored by Miller (1971) in a second experiment which involved a variation of the first. If the rate of presentation if the lists is slowed then new words should build up less quickly in short-term storage and so give the earliest words a much better chance to be transferred to long-term storage. This should be reflected in an enhanced elevation of the front part of the curve.

This effect has been shown in normal subjects by Glanzer and Cunitz (1966). It was also shown by the control group in Miller's experiment in which half the lists were presented at the original rate of $1\frac{1}{2}$ words per second. No such enhanced elevation of the first part of the curve was found in the demented group. If the dements' memory disorder was merely due to reduced capacity of the short-term store they would also have been able to benefit from the slower rate of presentation. That this benefit did not occur implies an additional difficulty and this could be the inability to establish new material in long-term storage.

Miller's (1971) experiments were taken to indicate a two-factor explanation of the memory disorder in dementia. It was hypothesized that there was both an impaired capacity of the short-term store and an additional difficulty in establishing new material in the long-term store. For a number of reasons, including the common problem in psychology that different types of experimental procedure often give results with rather different theoretical implications, it was decided to verify these conclusions.

The technique used was based on an experiment by Drachman and Arbit (1965) who were at that time investigating the memory disorder produced by bilateral mesial temporal lesions in man. Miller (1973) presented lists of words of increasing length in order to define each subject's 'word span'. The word span was defined as the longest list of words that the subject could repeat back accurately immediately after a single presentation. This was taken to represent the capacity of the short-term store and, as expected, it was significantly reduced in the demented group.

In the second part of the experiment supra-span learning was attempted. Each subject learned lists of words of length 'span + 1', 'span + 2', and 'span + 3' (the span here being defined as the individual subject's own word span). Each of these lists was presented against and again until either the subject was unable to give a correct recall of the list or 10 presentations had been reached. Since these lists were longer than the subject's own word span they would exceed the capacity of his short-term store and could therefore only be correctly recalled if part at least of the list had been passed into long-term storage. Undue difficulty in learning supra-span lists would indicate an impairment in getting new material into long-term storage. The results showed unequivocally that the demented group were markedly impaired as compared with the controls in learning supra-span lists.

Claiming that the capacity of the short-term store is reduced in dementia also poses the further question as to why this should be go. One possibility is that the absolute capacity is not reduced but that incoming material is coded less efficiently. It is obvious that any new material to be remembered is not stored in exactly the same way for as the subject hears or sees it, it must be transformed or 'coded' in such a way that it can be stored in memory. Inefficiently coded material is likely to take up more room in the short-term store and thus reduce the effective capacity of the store. The way in which memory systems code information at a physiological or biochemical level is not yet established but there is some indication from psychological experiments to indicate the features of words that may be abstracted for coding. If a group of words are all similar along a dimension used in coding within the short-term store, then they will be readily confused with one another and the list will be difficult to recall. Experiments on normal subjects using this principle have indicated that it is principally the acoustic characteristics of words that are coded in the short-term store (e.g., Baddeley, 1966a). The predominant nature of the acoustic characteristics of the words is demonstrated even when the words are presented to the subject visually.

Miller (1972b) based a study of coding in the short-term memory of demented subjects on the technique described by Baddeley (1966a). Subjects were presen-

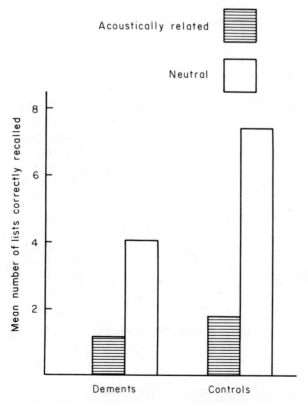

Figure 4. Recall of short lists of words as a function of acoustic similarity. Based on Miller (1972b)

54

ted with lists of four common words and were required to recall each list after a single presentation. Lists of acoustically similar (e.g., can, mat, man, cat), semantically similar (e.g., larger, great, huge, big), and unrelated words were used. No effect for semantically similar words was found in either group. Figure 4 shows that for both groups of subjects the number of correctly recalled lists was lower where the lists contained acoustically similar words than when they contained neutral words. This effect was significantly stronger in the control group and is assumed to reflect a more efficient level of coding by acoustic characteristics in the short-term stores of normal subjects. In other words this experiment supports the notion that inefficient coding could at least partly explain the lowered capacity of the short-term store in dementia.

Another possible reason for an apparently poor short-term memory in dementia is that the stage preceding it is faulty and does not allow an adequate input to the short-term store. There are no published accounts in the literature of experiments on iconic memory using demented subjects at the time of writing but some preliminary data obtained by Miller (1976) is of interest. In this experiment which used the backward masking technique, a row of six

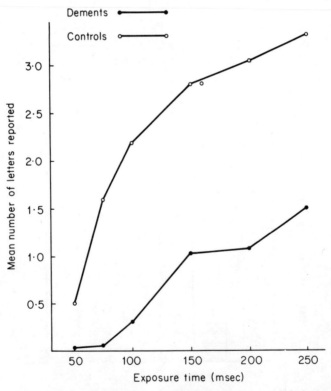

Figure 5. Number of letters reported from an array of six in a backward masking experiment

letters was presented tachistoscopically for a very brief time interval which varied between 50 and 250 milliseconds. Immediately following this stimulus came a random array of black and white squares to give a 'visual noise' effect and so mask any figural after effects. The subject's task is simply to report as many of the letters as he can. Figure 5 shows the relationship between the number of letters recalled and the exposure time. The demented group appear to require a longer exposure before they can start to report any of the letters with reliability and they are also unable to report as many letters for any exposure period above their threshold. Although this is only a preliminary investigation, and it would be unwise to rely too heavily upon its findings, it does suggest that this area is worth following up and that the memory impairment in dementia may originate from the very first stages of processing incoming information.

The remaining experiments in this series relate to the long-term component in the memory disorder associated with dementia. It was assumed at first that the problem was in getting material into long-term storage. This was very much in line with the general history of work in this field which was always oriented towards explanations in terms of impaired acquisition. However, there is nothing in the experiments of Miller (1971, 1973) to suggest that the long-term component of the memory disorder might not be due to other things, e.g. a relative inability to retrieve newly acquired information from the long-term store.

In recent years research into the severe memory disorders encountered in Korsakoff's syndrome and in patients with bilateral mesial temporal lesions has begun to impute these other aspects of the memory system including retrieval. In particular, Warrington and Weiskrantz (1970) described an experiment involving the long-term retention of lists of words. Whilst conventional tests of recall and recognition showed appreciable defects in their severely amnesic subjects, the presentation of partial information about the correct words at the time of recall brought the amnesic subjects' retention up to normal levels. In this case the partial information was either a visual display showing a fragmented version of the correct word (see the original report for an illustration of this) or the initial letter of the correct word. The occurrence of normal levels of retention when partial information was given at recall strongly suggests that the newly learned material has reached the long-term store and can be recalled if only the right type of cue is given. At least as far as the amnesic syndrome is concerned, this experiment shifts the emphasis from the acquisition of new material to its retrieval from memory.

The possibility that retrieval could also be an important factor in dementia led Miller (1975) to carry out an experiment similar to that of Warrington and Weiskrantz but using demented subjects. Subjects were required to read aloud and try to remember lists of 10 common words with each list being presented three times. Following a delay interval during which the subjects were distracted there was a test of retention. Three types of retention test were used. There were a straightforward recall, a recognition test in which the 10 correct words

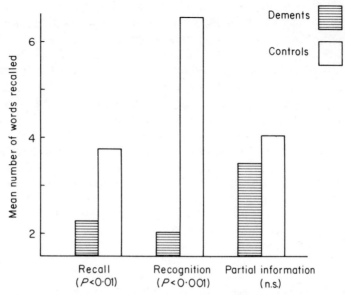

Figure 6. Retention of learned material as a function of different types of recall procedure. Based on Miller (1975)

were mixed with 10 incorrect words, and a partial information condition in which the initial letters of the correct words were supplied. Figure 6 summarizes the results and indicates large differences between the groups under the recall and recognition conditions. Both of these differences were statistically significant. There was no significant difference under the partial information condition.

If these results are accepted as indicating that the demented patient is able to establish new material in long-term storage but can only retrieve that information under special conditions, we must then go on to ask what it is that is peculiar about the retrieval process. Whatever it is that is involved probably only affects recently-acquired information since there is a strong clinical impression that patients recall distant events relatively well. Basically, two types of explanation can be presented although each is open to a number of variations. The demented patient may code new information in a bizarre way with the result that it can only be retrieved when the right kind of cue is available at recall. The alternative class of explanation implicates the actual retrieval process. One version put forward by Warrington and Weiskrantz (1970), with reference to their subjects with severe amnesia, is that the recall process becomes disinhibited. The subject fails to repress irrelevant information and is therefore in the position of recalling too much. Some incorrectly recalled words may even match alternatives supplied in recognition testing and thus give rise to erroneous positive recognitions. This explanation can therefore cope with the poor performance of the amnesic subjects on recognition testing.

It explains the much better performance when partial information is given on the grounds that the partial information limits the available choice of response without providing explicit alternatives that can be falsely matched with any incorrectly-recalled words. Further experiments by Warrington and Weiskrantz (1971) have failed to yield any evidence of unusual coding in amnesic subjects and, by implication, their 'disinhibition at recall' hypothesis is strengthened.

In considering these two types of explanation, let us first deal with the 'disinhibition at recall' hypothesis. A number of predictions can be derived from this hypothesis of which the simplest involves the free recall type of situation as used by Miller (1971). If the demented subject is disinhibited in recall he ought to produce at least as many words as the normal control in attempting to recall a list but should score badly because many of the words recalled are incorrect. It might be expected that the incorrect words would contain a high proportion of 'intrusions' from previous lists. Re-examination of the data from Miller

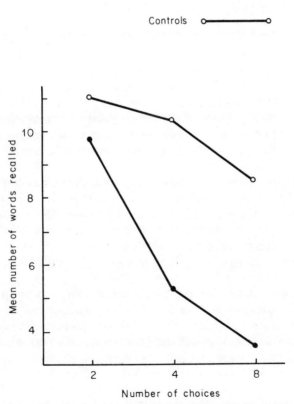

Figure 7. Performance on a recognition test as a function of the number of response alternatives. Based on Miller (1974b)

(1971) fails to confirm these expectations since the dements produced many fewer words than the controls when recalling the lists; neither was there a trend towards the dements giving a higher proportion of incorrect responses either in total or just when intrusions were considered.

A second prediction concerns the use of recognition testing. If dements suffer at recall because they tend to retrieve too many words, then increasing the number of alternatives in a recognition test should give greater opportunity for incorrect 'recognitions' to occur. This would exaggerate the normal tendency for performance on recognition tests to decline as a function of the number of response alternatives. Miller (1974b) got subjects to learn lists of words by a similar procedure to that used in the 1974 experiment. The only difference was that the lists contained 12 words instead of 10. In recognition testing the correct words were each set in an array of two, four, or eight words. The effect of altering the number of response alternatives on the accuracy of recognition is shown in Figure 7. Statistical analysis showed the groups by number of response-alternatives interaction to be significant thus confirming the prediction.

Although both positive and negative evidence has been obtained for the 'disinhibition at recall' hypothesis, no alternative explanation has yet received any support. Miller (1974b) did try to test the notion that the coding or organization of material in long-term storage might be at fault. The procedure was exactly the same as that described immediately above for the four alternative recognition conditions. For each correct word one of the alternatives was always semantically similar to it, a second was acoustically similar, and a third was unrelated. For example, if the correct word was 'jump', the semantically similar alternative might be 'leap', the acoustically similar word 'bump' and the neutral word 'house'. Since previous work with normal subjects had indicated that coding by semantic characteristics might be an important feature of long-term memory (Baddeley, 1966a; Baddeley and Dale, 1966), it was anticipated that where normal control subjects failed to choose the correct word they would tend to pick the semantically similar alternative. If long-term coding is disturbed in the demented subject, he would show either a weakened tendency in the same direction or would be likely to select a rather different kind of alternative when he failed to select the correct word. In fact no difference in the pattern of errors was found.

These results cannot be taken as definitely ruling out the possibility that dements use unusual methods of coding in long-term memory. The experiment described was not a particularly stringent test of this possibility and it is always possible that a more sensitive experimental design, or an experiment directed at other possible alternative methods of coding, might produce positive results. It is interesting in this context that Whitehead (1973a) has found that the type of error in recall produced by demented subjects is not the same as shown by those with depression.

As a final comment on the question of recall Whitehead's (1975) experiment is worth noting. She looked at the ability of dements to recognize which of

16 items (pictures or words) had been seen previously. Stimuli were either presented one at a time (with a 'yes' or 'no' response being required) or in a forced-choice format with one correct item being paired with an incorrect item. There was a trend towards better performance with the forced-choice format. An analysis of errors suggested that this was not because forced choice reduced the number of false positives (as would be implied by the disinhibition hypothesis) but because it elicited responses of which the subject was unsure. This result also implies that the readiness to respond when the subject is doutful is a factor that might need to be taken into account in future. However the conclusions drawn from this paper are weakened by the absence of a control group.

OTHER APPROACHES TO THE ANALYSIS OF MEMORY

Most of the experiments described above have obvious links with the sorts of experiment carried out by experimental psychologists interested in normal memory, and the individual investigations are each designed to look at a small part of the experimental process. An alternative way looking for the basis of the breakdown in memory has been suggested by Bevans (1972). Rather than using the piecemeal approach of experimental psychology, Bevans has attempted to gather a battery of tests derived more from the psycho-metric tradition that will measure different aspects of the memory process right through from attention to recall.

In the absence of any extensive data from Bevan's battery, it is impossible to say how effective this attempt will be in the analysis of the nature of the memory impairment. There are reasons which, to this writer at least, make this approach unlikely to offer anything that is any more worthwhile than the experimentally-oriented approach. Tests relating to very specific functions are difficult to design and are usually of doubtful validity. The analysis of profiles of test scores derived from a battery of tests that are inevitably intercorrelated also presents technical difficulties.

CONCLUSIONS AND COMMENTS

Within the study of the psychological manifestations of dementia, the topic of memory is almost unique in that systematic series of experiments have been carried out and there is at least an impression of a progression towards a better understanding of the issues involved. It is unfortunate that this progression appears to be towards a more and more complex picture of the memory disorder in dementia, with almost every conceivable aspect of the process of memory having been implicated at some time or other. It would be difficult to summarize this work succinctly and well nigh impossible to subsume all the findings under a single unifying principle. Rather than attempt either of these things we will just touch upon a few salient points.

With evidence pointing towards deficits at many points in the total memory process, work must proceed on a number of fronts. Most workers in the field of dementia stress the acquisition of new information and further analysis of this is required. It is certainly no longer sufficient just to suggest that short-term memory is impaired. Miller's experiments on coding within the short-term store and on iconic memory are a beginning but these studies need to be followed up and other hypotheses tested. Miller's later experiments also implicate the retrieval of information from the long-term store. Some confirmatory evidence would be useful here and, if obtained, ought to lead to further analyses of this aspect of the memory process.

Whilst it may be unsatisfactory for those with a strong desire for theoretical parsimony our present state of knowledge implies that explanations of the memory disorder in dementia are likely to be complex in that they will implicate a number of different aspects of the memory process. This is untidy but it is not surprising. Given that there is some relationship between anatomical regions of the brain and psychological functioning, and it need not be assumed that this is of a simple one-to-one variety, it is not unreasonable to assume that a degenerative process affecting most parts of the brain should result in impairments in most aspects of the complex functional system that constitutes memory.

On a final point, it could be argued with justification that the work discussed here is a biased sample of the available evidence relating to memory in dementia. The emphasis has undeniably been on verbal memory but the other material has been considered more appropriate for later chapters. The substantial amount of research with tests of learning and memory is reserved for Chapter 8, in which it can be set in the more appropriate context of diagnostic techniques. Such things as word learning tests may have diagnostic validity but they are not capable of sufficiently sophisticated theoretical analysis to contribute to the arguments advanced in the present chapter. It is accepted that conditioning is a topic which cannot be separated from memory in practical terms and consideration of the small amount of work on conditioning is reserved for the next chapter because it does not fit in well with the present emphasis on verbal learning and memory.

5
Other Psychological Findings in Dementia

The two previous chapters have reviewed the situation with regard to intellectual deterioration and memory changes in dementia. Whilst these two things form the most characteristic psychological disturbances that occur in dementia, a wide range of other psychological features have been reported. The involvement of language and personality can sometimes be quite striking and obvious from casual contact with the patient. On the other hand there are other, less immediately apparent, changes in such things as psychophysiological variables which can prove quite marked when the detailed investigations are carried out.

Once attention is directed away from the two major areas of intellectual decline and memory, there is much less concrete evidence on which to base opinions. As a result a number of sections in this rather heterogeneous chapter will be short and the discussion will not be able to match the inherent importance of the topics that are being discussed. If the reader emerges from this chapter with the impression that there are findings relating to many aspects of behaviour but little to link them up in any systematic way, then his impression will be an accurate picture of the present state of knowledge in these fields.

LANGUAGE

Disturbances in language are an important part of the total psychological change that occurs in dementia. They have been considered in some detail from a clinical point of view by Critchley (1964) and Stengel (1943, 1964). The first changes to be noticed are usually a general poverty of vocabulary and range of expression. The speech becomes concrete, circumlocutary and repetitive. It is of course difficult to distinguish these changes clearly from the general intellectual deterioration but definite dysphasic signs may also appear at some stage of the illness. There seems to have been no systematic examination of series of demented patients for different types of aphasic symptomatology other than that of Ernst *et al.* (1970a). These authors subjected a small group of demented patients to the system of examination of language functions described by Luria (1966). It was concluded that all showed poverty of vocabulary in narrative speech but, other than this, there was no general pattern of dysphasia. One feature that was common to several of the subjects was a difficulty in naming.

Disorders of naming are one of the few types of language disturbance in dementia that have been subjected to experimental analysis. Barker and Lawson (1968), and Lawson and Barker (1968) studied the ability of 100 subjects with senile dementia to name 24 objects and compared their performance with that of 40 age-matched normal controls. They recorded both the subject's ability to name the object correctly and the latency of the response if it was correct. As would be expected the dements had much greater difficulty in naming the objects but two other points of interest emerged. Although both groups of subjects were better at naming the more frequent words, whether in terms of latency or accuracy, the demented group were relatively much more handicapped when it came to producing the less-frequent words. The other difference between the groups was that demnostrating the use of the object enhanced the ability of the demented subject in naming but there was no similar effect for the control group.

Stengel (1964) has made the observation that the nominal dysphasia occurring in dementia is not like that occurring in aphasias due to other causes (i.e., focal lesions) in which the patient usually gives the strong impression that he knows what the object is but just cannot find the right word to apply to it. This notion has received support from the experiments of Rochford (1971). He compared the ability of patients with senile dementia to name objects with that of a rather younger group of subjects with dysphasia due to focal lesions. In attempting a rather subjective analysis of the type of error produced by the two groups, it appeared that in general the dysphasic group were failing to supply a name for an object that was correctly identified. In comparison, the dements failed to supply the correct name because they made errors in the recognition of the object. Their disability could thus be described as having an agnosic component.

In attempting to examine this hypothesis more closely Rochford argued that what was required was a naming task that reduced the problems involved in recognizing the object to be named. Such a task should benefit the demented but not the dysphasic group. Since the parts of the body are very familiar, and therefore easily recognized, subjects were asked to name these. As predicted the task gave considerable improvement in the naming of the demented group but made no difference to the performance of the dysphasics.

Even allowing for the question of recognition as revealed by Rochford's work, there possibly still remains a true difficulty in the production of words and Critchley (1964) has argued that the demented patient's poverty of speech is due to the inaccessibility of words in his vocabulary. Two further experiments bearing on this issue have been reported by Miller and Hague (1975). In the first of these, subjects with presenile dementia were given a version of Thurstone's (1938) word fluency test in which the subject has to give as many words beginning with the letter 'S' as he can in a 5-minute period. As compared with normal controls, the dements produced fewer words although in neither group was the cumulative total number of words reaching an asymptote by the end of the given time period. This suggests that both groups could have produced many more words if given a much longer time to do so.

The words produced by each subject were examined for their frequency of occurrence in normal usage according to the Thorndike and Lorge (1944) word count. It was found that the demented group produced a significantly lower proportion of the rarer words. It is tempting to argue that this shows that dements have a selective loss of the less common words in their vocabularies and also to link this with Barker and Lawson's (1968) finding that dements are impaired in naming objects when these have names that are less commonly encountered in everyday speech. Unfortunately further analysis of Miller and Hague's first experiment revealed a possible artifact. Normal subjects showed a definite tendency to produce very common words first and then go on to give the less common when some of the commoner ones had been exhausted. It could be argued that the demented group, being much slower to produce words, had simply not had time to get round to giving the less commonly used.

In order to examine this word frequency effect under conditions that would be free from any similar artifact, Miller and Hague (1975) went on to record a 2000-word sample of conversational speech from five presenile dements and five

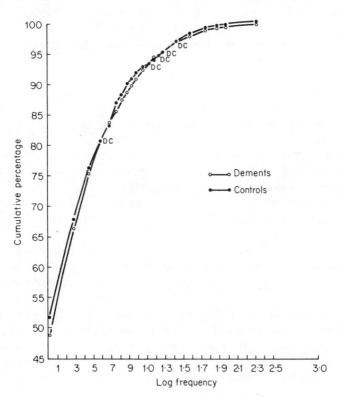

Figure 8. Cumulative percentage of words used as a function of their frequency of occurrence in the sample. From Miller and Hague *Psychological Medicine*, **5**, 255 (1975) by permission of the Editor of Psychological Medicine

control subjects. This recorded sample was then transcribed onto paper and the different words counted. It was thus possible to obtain for each subject the number of words used once in the sample, the number used twice, three times, etc. These were averaged across subjects in each group and graphed as the cumulative percentage of the total number of words against the logarithm of the word frequency. These graphs, which represent a derivation of Zipf's (1949) law, are shown in Figure 8. It can be seen that they give good approximations to straight lines for most of their range and it can be shown mathematically that the deviation from a straight line at the extremes is the consequence of sampling error.

The two curves shown in Figure 8 are almost identical. A general reduction in the availability of words would be reflected by a shift in the curve for the dements along the abscissa. A selective loss of the rarer words would have been indicated by an alteration in the slope of the straight line portion of the curves. There is obvious evidence for neither of these things although the caveat must be entered that these were very early cases (it would otherwise be difficult to collect the 2000-word sample of speech) and changes may occur later on in the disease process. Taking both of Miller and Hague's experiments together it seems that demented patients, at least in the early stages of the disease, have no loss of words from their vocabularies but they do exhibit a slowness in producing those words.

Another commonly reported feature of dementia is perseveration. Perseveration can be encountered in any aspects of behaviour but is usually most noticeable in speech. Freeman and Gathercole (1966) draw attention to three types of perseveration. The first, 'compulsive repetition' to use Luria's (1965) phrase, is where a response is repeatedly emitted. This type of perseveration is seen most often as a motor phenomenon, e.g. on being asked to put out his tongue the patient repeatedly puts it in and out. However, this type of perseveration can occur in speech where it is known as palilalia. The second type of perseveration can be understood as an 'impairment of switching', to use Luria's terminology again, and occurs when a response elicited by one stimulus is repeated inappropriately for a later stimulus. An example of this would be the patient who correctly names a watch and then describes the next object, say a pen, as a watch. Finally, there is ideational perseveration in which phrases and themes tend to appear again and again in the patient's spontaneous speech.

Freeman and Gathercole (1966) used a variety of verbal and non-verbal tasks designed to elicit the different types of perseveration and applied them to a group of patients with senile dementia and to a group of younger schizophrenics. Both groups showed a similar amount of perseveration when all types were considered together but the demented group produced a considerably larger number of perseverations of the type associated with impaired switching. There were no between-group differences in ideational perseveration but the schizophrenics made many more compulsive repetitions. This study provides an interesting indication of the type of perseveration to which dements may be most prone, but it cannot be considered definitive since the two groups differed appreciably in age and there was no normal control group. This study also offers no indication as to why the type of perseveration described as impaired switching occurs. The term 'impaired switching' implies one possible mechanism, but there are others and the alternatives need to be put to experimental test.

The receptive side of speech in dementia has been relatively neglected and it has only been possible to trace one experiment. This was based on a phenomenon known as the 'verbal transformation effect' which was first described by Warren and Gregory (1958). When a subject hears the same word or phrase presented over and over again (by recording a spoken version of the word on a closed tape loop and playing this continuously through a tape recorder) he is liable to report abrupt illusory changes in the stimulus. The subject may then briefly 'hear' other words or phrases. Obusek and Warren (1973) looked for this effect in two groups of elderly subjects one of which had 'senile deterioration', the other being normal. Their control group showed significantly more transformations but the transformations that were produced by the demented subjects involved more phonemic changes. In comparing these particular results with those of previous experiments by the same workers using very similar experimental conditions, the authors comment that the demented group behaved as if they were older than they really were in that the verbal transformation effect has been shown to decline with age. On the other hand the tendency to have more phonemic changes when a transformation does occur makes the dements look more like 10-year-old children. As Obusek and Warren are careful to point out, the conditions producing the verbal transformation effect are far removed from normal speech and this makes the implications of the present experiment difficult to assess.

The speech of demented patients does show disturbances, some of which are similar to those associated with dysphasia due to focal lesions. However closer examination shows that the character of these disturbances may not be identical in the two types of subject. Impairments in naming are common to both dysphasics with focal lesions and dements yet Rochford (1971) has shown that errors in naming may arise from different aspects of the total process involved in naming. Miller and Hague (1975) found no differences between demented and normal subjects in their analysis of word frequencies used in free speech, whilst Howes (1964) has shown that deviations from the normal pattern are typical in aphasia.

These differences between the language disorders found in dementia and those associated with subjects more traditionally regarded as being dysphasic (i.e., those with focal lesions) raise the semantic question as to whether the demented patient can be accurately described as having dysphasia. Since the total amount of research into language disorders in dementia is still quite small, especially where receptive disorders are concerned, any final answer to this question must wait until we have a much better understanding of the speech phenomena associated with dementia. ·

NEURO AND PSYCHOPHYSIOLOGICAL CHANGES

The principal neurophysiological changes in dementia have been reviewed by Levy (1969). With regard to the EEG the majority view is that the features in dementia are an accentuation of the changes produced by normal ageing. The alpha rhythm becomes more slowed than is usual for the normal elderly subject and there is greater diminution of the total amount of alpha activity. On the other hand, there are those like Hill and Driver (1962) who dispute this and claim that demented patients usually have EEGs that can be considered normal for their age.

There have been two studies that have repeatedly carried out EEG studies on demented patients. One of these, that of Letemendia and Pampiglioni (1958), obtained no change over a period of a year. Levy (1969) suggests that this failure to find change might be because the subjects used were advanced cases who might have passed their period of high rate of change. The second author to report serial EEGs was Gordon (1968) who found a definite deterioration in the EEGs of 10 of his 12 demented subjects over an interval varying between 9 months and 4 years.

One special type of EEG variable is the evoked potential or evoked response. This is shown by averaging the EEG response to a discrete stimulus over a very large number of trials. Levy et al. (1971) studied the somatosensory evoked potentials obtained from electrical pulses applied to the ulnar nerve. The general finding was that the latencies of the various peaks in the response were slower in patients with senile dementia as compared with lederly depressive patients of a similar age. In fact the discrimination between the two groups was good enough for the authors to press the potential value of the technique in differential diagnosis. The results of Levy et al. show a considerable parallel with those reported earlier by Straumanis et al. (1965). These authors used elderly patients diagnosed as having 'chronic brain syndromes' as their experimental subjects and found delays in the later components of visually evoked responses.

Another set of physiological measures which bear some relationship to brain functioning are those based on estimates of cerebral circulation and oxygen uptake in the brain. In general these functions have been found to be reduced in dementia (e.g., Hedlund et al., 1964). There also appears to be some relationship between these variables and measures based on the EEG. Obrist et al. (1963) found correlations between an index of EEG activity derived from the proportion of the record taken up by abnormal slow waves and a number of other variables, especially oxygen uptake.

Despite the popularity of the concept of arousal, there have been few attempts to use psychophysiological methods to assess the level of arousal in dementia. An almost isolated example is the investigation reported by Hemsi et al. (1968). These authors compared elderly dements with elderly depressed patients and predicted that the levels of arousal would be lower in the dements. They also expected that the arousal level would increase in successfully treated depressives but that it would decline with time in dements. They used two measures of arousal, the sedation and sleep threshold, and a measure of unstimulated salivation. The sleep threshold was higher in the depressed group thus confirming the notion of lower arousal levels in the dements, but no significant changes were found on re-testing with this measure. The results of the salivation measure were all non-significant but the trends were always contrary to the author's predictions.

The results of Hemsi *et al.* can be said to have raised more questions than they answer. One immediate problem facing this or any other experiment on arousal is that different measures or arousal are notorious for giving different results and therefore raising an immediate problem of interpretation. One aspect of the findings of Hemsi *et al.* has been confirmed in that Caird *et al.* (1963) were also able to obtain results suggesting lowered sedation and sleep thresholds in demented subjects. In view of the theories of dementia to be discussed later (Chapter Seven) further investigations of arousal level in dementia would be useful.

The influence of dementia on the peripheral nervous system has not received much attention but there are some experiments on peripheral nerve conduction. The most important study here is that of Levy *et al.* (1970) who set out to confirm and extend an earlier finding by Levy and Poole (1966). This was that patients with senile dementia had a significant retardation in the conduction of impulses along peripheral motor nerves. Levy *et al.* had 28 patients with senile dementia and 19 controls who were patients with a similar age range and who had functional psychiatric disorders. The demented group was found to have a lower mean motor nerve conduction velocity but the difference between the groups failed to reach an acceptable level of statistical significance. However, it was noted that an independent assessment of the subjects using a dementia rating scale had produced high scores for some of the control group with the possible implication that some of them might have been misclassified. There was a significant correlation of -0.51 between conduction velocity and the score on the dementia rating scale, and when subjects with high scores on this scale were compared with those who had low scores there was a significant difference in conduction velocity. Nine of the original demented group were retested a year later and all three of those for whom the score on the dementia rating scale had increased also showed a further slowing of motor nerve conduction velocity.

There is very little in the way of general conclusions that can be drawn concerning these physiological findings. The slowing of motor nerve conduction and the changes in evoked responses suggest that a general slowing of activity takes place throughout the whole of the nervous system. The *EEG* observations could also be interpreted as being in line with this conclusion. The extent of the neuro- or psycho-physiological changes occurring in dementia and the degree to which they might be subsumed under some general interpretation, like that of a slowing of nervous activity or a reduction in arousal levels, is undecided. The whole area requires further elucidation.

CONDITIONING AND LEARNING

Terms like 'conditioning', 'learning', and 'memory' have a considerable semantic overlap. 'Conditioning' usually refers to certain kinds of simple learning situations and 'learning' is difficult to disentangle from 'memory' operationally because the two things are so interrelated. Commonly the term 'memory' is used by experimental psychologists to refer to the study of verbal learning and memory using certain relatively well defined experimental procedures. As far as 'memory' in this sense is concerned, the relevant material was dealt within Chapter Four. This section includes everything else that might be subsumed under these labels.

The number of reported experiments has been small. In general the experimental procedures have not been described very well, thus making the reader rather over dependent upon the authors' interpretation of their data. Both Brown *et al.* (1960) and Solyom and Barik (1965) have followed the classical conditioning paradigm. Brown *et al.* used a technique devised by Gantt (1950) whereby the psychogalvanic response and changes in respiration are used as the conditioned response to both visual and auditory conditioned stimuli preceding the electric shock which acts as the unconditioned stimulus. Subjects indicated by the report to be almost certainly demented showed lower rates of both types of conditioned response. They were also less responsive in their unconditioned reactions to the shock and this could at least partly explain their apparently poorer conditioning.

Solyom and Barik (1965) utilized classical eye-blink conditioning (the conditional stimulus being a tone which is paired with a puff of air to the eye thus eliciting a blink). Their demented subjects were slower than elderly normals in acquiring the conditioned response. Unlike the experiment of Brown *et al.*, the results did not show the demented group to have a lower level of responsivity than their age-matched controls, although both the elderly groups were less responsive than younger normal subjects.

Kiev *et al.* (1962) also showed that subjects with diffuse cerebral atrophy were slower to condition in an instrumental avoidance situation in which the electric shock following the conditioned stimulus could be avoided by making an appropriate motor response. These subjects showed a relatively greater impairment in conditioning as the task was made more complex by using more than one conditioned stimulus and requiring a differential response according to the nature of the stimulus.

Despite its obvious potential value in the management of demented patients (see Chapter Nine), there has been very little research into the basic operant conditioning procedures. Mackay (1965) looked at lever pulling for different reinforcements (money, cigarettes or chocolate) and under different reinforcement schedules. Elderly control subjects developed patterns of responding very similar to those occurring in other human and animal studies. In contrast, the demented group (defined operationally in terms of memory impairment) gave much lower, more erratic, response rates and were not sensitive to changes in reinforcement contingencies. Mackay's experiments suggest that the poor classical conditioning found by the authors cited above is matched by even worse operant conditioning. They also imply the pessimistic conclusion that the behaviour of demented patients will be refractory to modification by operant techniques.

Mackay's work has been followed up by Ankus (1970) and Ankus and Quarrington (1972). They used a similar human analogue of the animal Skinner Box situation to that of Mackay, and subjects were again required to pull a lever for a reward. Suggesting that appropriateness of reinforcement might be a crucial factor they used both money and the subjects' own choice of fluid as reinforcers. Within demented subjects females did better with the monetary reward but males preferred fluids. The key finding was that, given the correct reinforcer, subjects conditioned well and were also shown to be very sensitive to alterations in the schedules of reinforcement in exactly the same way as the normal controls.

Demented patients have definitely been shown to be impaired in both classical and operant conditioning. In the case of operant conditioning this is far from being due entirely to a failure to condition as when appropriate reinforcers are given good patterns of performance can be obtained. It is less clear whether the poorer classical conditioning can be explained in similar terms. Simple conditioning and verbal learning and memory by no means exhaust all the possibilities for research in·learning and memory. It is regrettable that there has been no work on the learning and retention of complex non-verbal behaviour and so there is little but idle speculation that could be offered.

PERSONALITY

Clinicians have given accounts of changes in personality as a consequence of dementia and these descriptions were summarized in the introductory chapter. Briefly, the most common change is thought to be an exaggeration of the patient's premorbid traits, whilst some patients are thought to reverse their personality characteristics. These can only be regarded as the features occurring early on in the illness. With the steady progressive deterioration in all aspects of psychological functioning, the ultimate picture is that of apathy and inertia with a flattening of all aspects of the personality.

The measurement of personality change is notoriously difficult. Projective tests like the Rorschach and Thematic Apperception Test are in common use and have been used in the study of dementia. Whilst the advocates of projective tests may have considerable faith in their value, their poor validity as assessed by objective methods makes the results obtained from them of little value for the more sceptical observer. Personality questionnaires are better established as scientific tools but are still rather insensitive instruments for the assessment of change. They also present problems when used with older populations. Questionnaires are almost invariably developed on young adult subjects and, even within this limited age range, they may be drawn from an unrepresentative population such as students. The transfer of these tests to older people may mean that the norms are invalid, and Gilmore (1972) has shown that older subjects do not always have the same understanding of the items as younger subjects. Other methods of assessing personality, such as the so-called 'objective methods' (Cattell, 1965), have not been used with older subjects and need not concern us here.

Rorschach himself was the first person to describe the application of his inkblot technique to patients with senile dementia (Rorschach, 1942). Other investigators have obtained remarkably consistent results (Ames et al., 1954; Dorken and Kral, 1951; Orme, 1955) in terms of the various measures commonly derived from Rorschach protocols. Rorschach interpreted his findings as showing 'egocentric extrasensitivity' where 'extrasensitivity' has much in common with the usual meanings attached to 'extraversion'. Other interpretations mention such things as disinhibition and a loss of the finer nuances of personality (Dorken and Kral, 1951) or reduced insight and lowered awareness of inner conflicts (Orme, 1955).

There are very few studies of demented populations using personality questionnaires. With regard to the Minnesota Multiphasic Personality Inventory, Uecker (1969) compared two methods of administering this scale to elderly demented patients. He found test–re-test reliabilities that were lowered to such a degree that he concluded that the use of this scale was not justified with such populations. On the Maudsley Personality Inventory, elderly demented subjects appeared to have higher levels of neuroticism than normal subjects (Bolton, 1967). However, these two groups did not differ in extraversion, a finding which is in conflict with Rorschach's (1942) analysis.

Patients with dementia have sometimes been described as being apathetic and poorly motivated. In trying to get these impressions onto a sounder basis, Katz et al. (1960) carried out a complete neurological, psychiatric, psychological and social evaluation of a very large sample. Contrary to the common prejudice, they concluded that their demented subjects were moderately well motivated and interested during interviews and psychological testing. There was no obvious relationship between motivation and level of intellectual impairment. Many of the sample responded in an adaptive way to stress although there were some whose behaviour became grossly disorganized and gave catastrophic reactions. In this context stress was considered to be produced by failure on such things as intelligence test items and it is possible that some subjects responded well because they did not see this sort of thing as being particularly stressful.

It is obvious to all who are familiar with demented patients that marked changes do occur in personality. Unfortunately there is little in the way of useful data that would allow this statement to be elaborated upon. Savage (1973) appears to think that what is required to remedy this situation is more data. The difficulties in the use of presently available techniques with aged and demented subjects as highlighted by Gilmore (1972) and Uecker (1969) imply that what will be required are more-appropriate techniques rather than more data from the techniques already in use.

MISCELLANEOUS

The presentation so far has by no means exhausted the possible range of psychological disturbances in dementia. Investigations of other aspects of behaviour are extremely rare and all that might be available for potentially important areas are one or two extremely inadequate studies.

Perception

Perceptual disturbances are probably present in dementia (Williams, 1956a). There have also been some neuropsychological investigations with a bearing on the topic of perception. Willanger and ·Klee (1966) discovered that despite any abnormality of ocular movement, 13 of a total sample of 300 cases of cerebral atrophy showed visual disturbances when asked to fixate on a particular object. Waviness of the linear contours and diplopia were the most common abnormalities, and there was the occasional incidence of a reported change in the apparent size of the object. The fact that just over half of this particular sub-group had had closed head injuries in the past raises doubts as to whether these findings really are characteristic of dementia.

Another investigation which was concerned to some extent with perceptual processes was that of Ernst et al. (1970b) who examined nine cases of presenile dementia for gnostic and praxic disturbances. A variety of changes occurred on the gnostic tests but with no characteristic pattern of impairment. There was similarly no clear type of apraxia although ideomotor apraxia and apraxia for dressing emerged as being the most common. The only study of auditory perception known to this author is that of Obusek and Warren (1973) on the verbal transformation effect which was discussed in the section on language.

Spatial Ability

In view of the general demonstration that performance IQ is lower than verbal IQ in dementia (see Chapter Three) spatial disturbances might be expected. Williams (1956b) tested 60 patients with senile dementia using paper and pencil mazes. These subjects performed very badly although they did show an improvement with repeated testing. Unfortunately the absence of a control group makes this experiment difficult to interpret.

Other evidence of spatial disturbances has been found by Ajuriaguerra et al. (1968) and Gaillard (1970). The latter claimed a disintegration of the body schema in dementia based on the fact that demented subjects were unable to fit together pictures of different parts of the human body to make a whole. Ajuriaguerra et al. (1966) looked at their subjects' appreciation of mirror images and found a loss of the ability to appreciate reflected space. For example, an elderly demented subject seeing an object situated over his left shoulder through a mirror would reach through the mirror to get it.

Information Processing

Hibbard *et al.* (1975) used information theory measures in looking at the ability of subjects to make certain types of sensory discrimination. The results showed that normal elderly subjects achieved lower scores on a measure of transmitted information but a demented group did even worse. This paper appears to be unique within the field of dementia in its use of information theory. Since information theory yields a powerful technique for quantifying performance on very simple tasks it could be of great value in the study of dementia where the more advanced cases can only perform adequately in the easiest of experimental situations.

Distractability

This is often alledged to be a characteristic of many types of 'brain damaged' subjects and there is evidence that demented patients can also be distractible. Lawson *et al.* (1967) required their subjects to report back sets of digits presented auditorily or visually. On some trials this was done against a background of distracting stimuli, e.g. the key digits were read by a female voice with a further set of digits ready by a male voice as the distractor. In the visual condition the distracting digits were presented in the wrong colour. As compared with normals patients, with presenile dementia where significantly more distracted in the auditory modality but not in the visual modality. This does not necessarily prove a modality difference in the effects of distraction as the distracting conditions used in the two modalities were not matched for their potency as distractors.

Motor Skills

A final aspect of behaviour that has been studied is that of psychomotor performance. Birren and Botwinick (1951) showed that writing speed was significantly reduced in senile dementia. The task used was simply that of copying a random series of digits or a random series of words as quickly as possible. The authors tentatively suggest that this retardation in writing is due more to changes of an aphasic nature rather than a reduction in motor speed.

That true motor changes do occur is implied by the description by Pearce and Miller (1973) of extrapyramidal changes (tremor, rigidity, etc.) in presenile dementia, and Ajuriaguerra *et al.* (1966) demonstrated ideomotor apraxia in some cases of senile dementia. Further experimental evidence comes from Miller (1974a) who showed that patients with presenile dementia were much slower than age-matched normal controls on a simple peg-board task. This merely required the subject to move 10 pegs from one set of holes to another and could not have been confounded by dysphasia in the way that Birren and Botwinick's (1951) experiment was.

Assuming that a retardation in motor speed does occur it is possible that this might arise in at least two ways. The demented subject could be slow in actually executing movements or he could be slow in deciding when or where to move. This was further examined by Miller (1974a) using an experimental procedure based on that devised by Singleton (1954) to study the effects of normal ageing on motor speed. The apparatus consisted of five channels set in a horizontal board and radiating from a central point. According to the indications given by lights in a separate display, the subject moved a stylus from the centre down one of the channels and back to the centre to start the next trial. Timers recorded the time spent at the central point deciding where to move after the appropriate signal had appeared and the actual time taken to execute the movement. Results showed the demented group to be much slower than the controls in the execution of the movements. The difference in decision times was of a much lower order. This contrasts with studies of the effects of normal ageing where the main difference is in decision times. The observed retardation in the execution of this relatively simple movement was also much larger than could be accounted for by any of the reported delays in motor nerve conduction (Levy et al., 1970; Levy and Poole, 1966).

GENERAL COMMENT

The topics covered in this chapter have necessarily been very diverse and there has been very little in the way of a unifying theme. What does seem to emerge from this and the previous two chapters is that whatever aspect of behaviour we care to look at, the demented patient is likely to show some change. This is hardly surprising because of the intimate relationship between the brain and psychological functioning and the fact that the pathological changes in dementia are so diffusely dispersed within the brain. Another obvious conclusion is that many potentially interesting and important aspects of the psychopathology of dementia have been almost totally neglected. For example, the appreciation of spatial relationships and motor skills are important in many everyday tasks essential to independent living and yet there is no systematic research in these areas. The available information comes from a handful of scattered investigations most of which are far from being of the highest quality.

As with the case of the changes produced by normal ageing there is a temptation to try to reduce all the varied phenomena to being the consequence of a single variable such as poor motivation. There are no published investigations of experiments specifically concerned with the effects of manipulating motivation in demented subjects, although Katz et al. (1960) concluded from their clinical observations that demented patients did not necessarily have impaired motivation. Furthermore the wide range of experiments that have found differential effects in which one variable is affected to a much greater degree than another also argue against the use of a single underlying variable such as motivation to explain all the behavioural changes in dementia. Again, as was the case with motivation as a possible explanation of the changes associated with normal ageing, there is no denying that poor motivation might not be a contributory factor in some observed changes. We are merely denying that it is a convincing total explanation.

6

The Relationship Between Psychological and Other Variables

The previous chapters have presented a wide range of psychological disturbances that have been found in association with dementia. It is to be expected that these psychological changes will bear some relationship to other, more physical variables, pathological, radiological, etc., that are known to reflect the state of the brain in dementia. Many investigators have attempted to look for such correlations and a number have failed to find them. As we shall see in the following chapter this failure has led some to the drawing of rather dubious conclusions about the causal factors in dementia. This is because it can be argued that if the psychological changes in dementia are not correlated with the claimed physical changes, then the latter are unlikely to be the cause of the former.

A basic problem is that for a variety of reasons, correlations between psychological measures on the one hand and pathological, radiological, and other physical variables on the other, are not likely to be very large. Because of this only well-designed studies that are sensitive enough to detect small correlations are likely to show positive findings. Before attempting to evaluate the evidence it is essential to consider the methodological problems in some detail.

METHODOLOGICAL ISSUES

The magnitude of a correlation between two variables can be affected by a number of things. Most of these will tend to weaken the calculated correlation coefficient. Measures that are unreliable (in the technical sense of containing a lot of error variance, i.e. not being very accurate) cannot correlate together to a high degree. To put this in another way, in psychometric theory reliability is assessed by means of the extent to which a given measure will correlate with itself on repeated application to the same group of subjects. It is intuitively obvious that a measure that does not correlate well with itself can hardly be expected to correlate any better with a second variable. Unfortunately, it is the case that many of the measures used in the investigations to be discussed in this chapter are such as to be likely to have low reliability. Many psychological measures have levels of reliability below that which might reasonably be desired and it is doubtful if some of the non-psychological measures, such as those based on the air encephalogram or the various neurophysiological parameters, would fare much better.

Another source of influence that may depress the correlation is where one of the variables is partly determined by a third, independent factor. The most important independent factor here is the premorbid level of the particular variables that are being examined. As an example consider a psychological variable like IQ. The IQs of a group of demented patients are likely to have shown wide variation in premorbid level. The effects of the illness will be to depress the subjects' IQs but these IQs will still, in part, reflect premorbid levels in that a person with a high IQ may well show appreciable deterioration and yet remain near or about the premorbid level of an initially less well endowed subject. In theory, a correlation could be corrected to eliminate the effect of different premorbid levels amongst the subjects but since these premorbid levels are rarely known this has never proved possible in practice.

There are other methodological difficulties liable to result in attentuated correlations which need not be elaborated in detail. Any relationship between the two types of variables may not be a simple linear one and so may not be adequately expressed by a conventional correlation coefficient. None of the published investigations appears to have considered this possibility for which some appropriate statistical procedures do exist. Another difficulty arises because some of the things with which psychological measures can be correlated are not simple variables. A large number of scores can be derived from the air encephalogram, electroencephalogram, etc., and there is often no *a priori* reason for deciding which of the range of possibilities might best be related to psychological functions. Finally, high correlations are most easily obtained where the subjects show a wide range of scores on the two variables. It is especially the case with the psychological variables that demented subjects tend to be massed at the lower end of the scale.

These difficulties are more than sufficient to justify the original assertion that any true association between psychological and non-psychological variables is not going to result in a high calculated correlation coefficient when looked for in practice. Only research strategies liable to be sensitive to low correlations are likely to produce significant results. Since most of the published evidence is based on unreliable measures applied to relatively small numbers of subjects, an inability to show a statistically significant correlation cannot be taken as a powerful argument that no real association exists. Only after highly sensitive experimental designs have failed to reject the null hypothesis can we afford to forget the very real possibility that the experimental design was just not good enough.

AIR ENCEPHALOGRAPHY

Since patients with suspected dementia, especially if in the presenium, are often investigated by air encephalography (AEG) an obvious set of possible correlations are those between psychological factors and the various measures that can be derived from the AEG. For those unfamiliar with this radiological technique a brief description is in order.

The aim of the technique is to outline the ventricles and certain other cavities in and around the brain. Normally cerebrospinal fluid (CSF) is generated within the ventricles and this both fills the ventricles and circulates round the brain and spinal cord. Because CSF has the same low degree of radio opacity as brain tissue the ventricles are not outlined in a straight X-ray of the head. In order that the ventricles can be seen a radio opaque substance, in this case air, must be introduced into the ventricles. This is done by making a lumbar puncture, drawing off some CSF, and injecting about 30. ml of air. Since air tends to rise it can be manipulated into the ventricles and these are outlined in the resulting X-ray. Such an AEG from a demented patient is shown in the Frontispiece. In this picture the two lateral ventricles and the third ventricle are clearly outlined. They are much larger than would be the case for a normal person. The small dark patches beneath the skull show that a degree of cortical atrophy has enabled air to circulate over the surface of the brain and to outline some of the widened sulci.

Many different measures can be derived from features in the AEG and some of the more commonly used ones are shown diagrammatically in Figure 9. Apart from the problem of determining the best measures to use there are a number of technical difficulties in taking measurements from the AEG. For example, slight alterations in the positioning of the head when the film is taken can alter the measurements. The distance between the X-ray source, the patient's head and the plate are also critical and cannot always be controlled with the greatest accuracy. Bull (1961) and Nielsen et al. (1966) give detailed discussions of these problems.

Despite the difficulties involved, most investigators seem to have found a positive relationship between the degree of atrophy as revealed by the AEG and clinical and/or psychological changes. One of the few negative instances is Lindgren (1951) who failed to find any close relationship between mental changes and the appearance of the AEG. McCormick (1962) also claimed to find little evidence of any relationship between various measures taken from the AEG and ratings of the degree of dementia in 37 patients over the age of 60 years. However, McCormick's report, being a dissertation, does provide more of the raw data than is usual in a published report, and by using this data the present writer was able to show a statistically significant relationship between the widths of the anterior horns and the ratings of dementia.

It is unfortunate that most of the positive evidence comes from investigations in which the level of ratiological sophistication has been in excess of that used in the measurement of psychological change. The latter has often consisted of poorly described clinical ratings which may or may not have been made independently of the evaluation of the AEG. Positive associations between various AEG indices of atrophy and ratings of such things as degree of dementia, memory deterioration, and social competence have been claimed by Burhenne and Davies (1963), Engeset and Lonnum (1958) and Kiev et al. (1962). The experiment of Kiev et al. is of particular interest from a psychological point of view because, within their group of 19 subjects with progressive dementia,

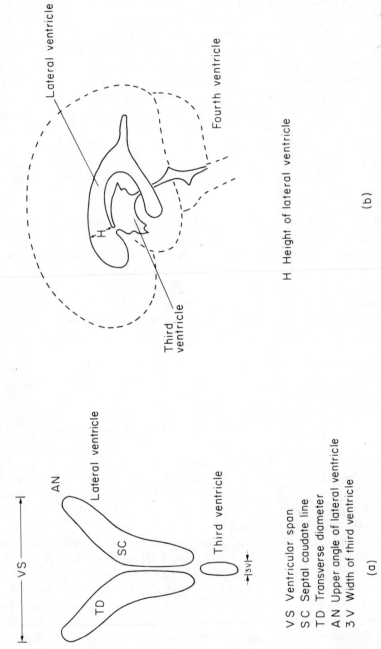

Lateral ventricle

Fourth ventricle

Third ventricle

H Height of lateral ventricle

(b)

AN

Lateral ventricle

VS

SC

TD

Third ventricle

3V

(a)

VS Ventricular span
SC Septal caudate line
TD Transverse diameter
AN Upper angle of lateral ventricle
3V Width of third ventricle

Figure 9. Outlines of the cerebral ventricles as seem in (a) anteroposterior and (b) lateral views. Some of the measurements that can be derived from the AEG are indicated

there was an inverse relationship between the degree of atrophy and the speed of learning of an instrumental avoidance task.

A rather better investigation is that of Gosling (1955) who traced 68 cases of dementia over the age of 45 years who had been seen at the National Hospital for Nervous Diseases in London and for whom an AEG had been carried out. Only 10 cases failed to show atrophy on the AEG. When reference was made to ratings of the degree of dementia as slight, moderate, or marked, all but two of this subgroup of 10 were considered to have only slight dementia (within the total sample 27 were rated as having a slight degree of dementia). Six of the ten cases without radiologically demonstrated atrophy were followed up and only one showed progressive deterioration which implies the possibility of misdiagnosis in this subgroup. Overall the relationship between the rated degree of dementia and the incidence of appearances of atrophy on the AEG reached a high level of statistical significance.

Gosling also comments on a number of other cases with radiological signs of atrophy but who had no clinical evidence of dementia. This phenomenon also arises in the later paper of Mann (1973). Mann traced 49 out of 54 patients from the hospitals associated with the Institute of Psychiatry in London, with reported cerebral atrophy on the basis of AEGs carried out between 1962 and 1966. Of the 49, only 33 were discharged from hospital with a diagnosis of dementia and 29 of these had died at follow-up around 7 years later. Of those that were dead, the majority had died with clear evidence of advanced dementia. None of those that were alive at follow-up showed any current evidence of dementia nor was there any convincing evidence of a decline in measured IQ. It is interesting to note that, despite the absence of dementia at follow-up, the survivors had a high level of psychiatric morbidity in general. One implication of this is that a radiological picture suggestive of atrophy is not a guarantee of dementia as determined on other grounds.

Sjaasted and Lonnum (1966) specifically examined the long-term prognosis of patients with demonstrated enlargement of the ventricles. In general, ventricular enlargement was associated with a much higher mortality rate than would be expected from a normal population of a similar age. In those who survived in their sample, there was a tendency towards a deterioration in clinical and occupational levels. Sjaasted and Lonnum's subjects included patients whose ventricular enlargement was due to progressive cerebral disease (such as the dementias) and these had a worse prognosis than those whose enlargement was due to such causes as a temporary increase in intracranial pressure where there was a little or no tendency to progression in the underlying pathology. Almost all of those managing to remain at work over a mean follow-up period of 6·5 years were in this latter category.

The AEG studies cited so far have almost invariably used rather global assessments of intellectual functioning often based upon unreliable forms of measurement like clinical ratings. There are a small number of reports of studies that have used rather more sophisticated assessments of psychological variables. Not only have they used better measures but they have also examined a wider variety of psychological functions.

There are two major studies in this category but before going on to describe these, the smaller investigation of McFie (1960) ought to be mentioned. McFie correlated linear measurements of the cella media taken from the AEG with psychometric data from the Wechsler Bellevue Intelligence Scale in 51 subjects. He found a significant correlation between the radiological measure and intellectual deterioration as given by the Wechsler deterioration index. This index is alleged to measure the amount of intellectual deterioration but it is unfortunate that, as will be argued in Chapter Eight, the index has rather poor validity.

The first of the major studies referred to above is that of Matthews and Booker (1972). Their report deals with a total sample of 97 subjects drawn from patients with a wide variety of neurological conditions, only some of which could be regarded as falling within the category of dementia as defined in this book. The mean age of the subjects was also low in comparison with the usual age ranges associated with presenile dementia. Nevertheless this investigation is of some interest in the present context since it is one of very few to compare AEG findings with a range of adequately specified and measured psychological functions.

A wide range of measures derived from the AEG were considered together with scores from 24 different psychological variables. The latter were intended to measure abstraction ability, motor and sensory performance, as well as intelligence as measured by the Wechsler Adult Intelligence Scale. The main comparison of interest is between two subgroups of 15 subjects, each selected from the top and bottom thirds of the distribution of subjects according to the total size of the ventricles as measured by planimeter. The relatively small size of the two groups as compared to the total subject population was because of the necessity to control for age which had been shown to be related to ventricular size.

Of the 24 different psychological measures, all but three showed a lower level of performance for the group with the larger ventricular system. Statistical analysis only showed six of the measures with a trend in the expected direction to have a significant between-groups difference. Using so many measures, one or two might have been expected to show a statistically 'significant' difference on the basis of chance alone but six is too many to be explained in this way. Those that were significant consisted of two measures of performance on a pencil maze, the Halstead category test, speed of movement on the pegboard task, the speed of recognizing forms placed on the hand by stereognosis, and a measure of finger agnosia.

Unfortunately these measures have no obvious characteristic in common. On the intelligence test the only appreciable trend was towards a higher performance IQ in the group with smaller ventricles ($P = 0.10$). For those tests, like the sensory and motor tests, that could be applied to either hand there was a general trend for performance to be worse on the side contralateral to the hemisphere of the brain having greatest evidence of cerebral atrophy.

By far the most extensive work in this area is that of Willanger and his associates. This is recorded in a number of publications (Willanger, 1970a, b; Willanger *et al.*, 1968) which all seem to relate to the same large series of radiologically investigated patients. Because of this Willanger's work will be described as a whole without further differentiation between the individual accounts. The basis of this work was provided by a large series of 300 unselected patients subjected to AEG and psychological testing in a Copenhagen hospital. As in the previously described work of Matthews and Booker (1972), the subjects came from a wide age range covering the whole span of adult life and their diagnoses were not confined to the dementing diseases of most relevance in the present context. Nevertheless a substantial proportion of subjects do seem to have had dementia in the sense that it is used in this book. A wide variety of procedures were used in the psychological examinations although not all seem to have been applied to every subject. Hence the specific findings were often based on samples well below the maximum size of 300.

Willanger's findings can be summarized as showing that the subjects with the lowest degree of atrophy, as ascertained from the AEG, tended to be those with the fewest spontaneous complaints of reduction in functioning and the best test performances. Those with severe atrophy performed badly on the psychological tests and were often too impaired to give a reasonable account of their functioning. In general, better correlations between radiological and psychological measures were obtained by using indices of cortical atrophy than by using assessments of ventricular enlargement. The highest correlations came from the use of a total atrophy score which was based on both the cortical and ventricular components. As in the case with Matthews and Booker (1972), there was a relationship between age and the indices of atrophy such that older subjects tended to have greater atrophy. However, the correlations with psychological variables generally remained even within subgroups which were relatively homogeneous for age. The specific tests which correlated with the radiological variables included a paired associate learning test, a sorting test based on the Hanfmann–Kasanin Concept Formation Test, the Goldstein–Scheerer Cube Test, and assessments of intellectual impairment based on the results of the Wechsler Adult Intelligence Scale.

As a whole, work on the relationship between the AEG and psychological variables raises a number of questions. The case for some degree of correlation between the two types of measure seems to be well established but the details need to be worked out. Cognitive functioning appears to decline as atrophy increases but there is no consistent information as to what aspects of cognitive functioning show the best relationship. Probably it is expecting too much to ask for this information before the exact nature of the intellectual decline in dementia is better understood. Because the changes in memory are better understood, and can be measured with a useful degree of accuracy, it is a pity that performance on memory tests has not been more frequently related to the AEG.

A further issue is the nature of the most predictive features of the AEG as far as psychological changes are concerned. These may well vary with the nature of the psychological function involved but there is some controversy with respect to intellectual changes. Both Gosling (1955) and Mann (1973) agree that the size of the ventricles is important and the same conclusion can be drawn from the data presented by McCormick (1962). Gosling also considers that the width of the sulci are of significance but Mann disagrees with this. On the other hand, the work of Willanger and his associates indicates that, whilst a total atrophy measure based upon both cortical and ventricular components comes out best, the signs of cortical atrophy are more predictive than those of ventricular enlargement. This problem remains to be resolved but the more heterogeneous nature of Willanger's subjects may be of some significance as may the variation between experiments in the methods of estimating intellectual deterioration.

What is required are more investigations that are both radiologically and psychologically sophisticated. It is unfortunate that so far the most psychologically sophisticated reports are those, like Willanger's, which are based on subjects with a variety of clinical conditions.

NEUROPATHOLOGICAL CHANGES

In Chapter One, certain neurophathological changes were described as occurring in dementia. These can now be examined in relationship to psychological changes. There is an immediate difficulty in this. Usually neuropathological findings only become available after death and the demented patient is often inaccessible to psychological investigation during the terminal stages of his illness. Thus the behavioural features must be assessed some time before death and presumably whilst the neuropathological changes are still in progress. The alternative is to rely on biopsy samples taken near the time of psychological examination. The use of biopsy specimens is complicated by the problem of sampling within the brain where neuropathological changes may not be evenly spread. Furthermore brain biopsies are very rarely considered justified on ethical grounds. In the small number of published reports all appear to have correlated intellectual changes in life with pathological findings after death and it is difficult to decide from the accounts how long before death the assessments were made.

Grünthal (1926) was possibly the first to look at neuropathological data in this way. He classified cases of Alzheimer's disease as mild, moderate, or severe in their degree of mental impairment. These classifications were then related to a variety of histological changes and Grünthal claimed that there was a close association between the two sets of data.

A series of papers by Rothschild (Rothschild, 1937, 1942; Rothschild and Sharp, 1941) claimed that there was no evidence of any relationship between psychological and neuropathological changes. In separate groups of subjects with both senile and arteriosclerotic dementia, Rothschild (1937 and 1942) was able to find no correlation between pathological features (loss of cells, senile plaques, neurofibrillary tangles, etc.) and the degree of intellectual deterioration. Rothschild carried out no statistical analyses but the 1937 paper does give all the raw data. The present writer could find no way of analysing the data to show a statistically significant correlation.

Bearing in mind the methodological comments made in the introduction to this chapter Rothschild's experiments were not carried out in such a way as to be likely to produce significant results. The groups were not very large in size and the nature of the intellectual assessments was not described. These were almost certainly only based on clinical impressions. (To be fair, the same criticisms could also be made of Grünthal's (1926) paper which produced the claimed 'close correlation'.) One may hazard a guess that the two sets of data in Rothschild's investigations were not obtained independently.

Rothschild's third paper (Rothschild and Sharp, 1941) presents a small series of individual case studies which are designed to make the point that mild degrees of neuropathological involvement may be associated with marked clinical dementia and more severe pathological features with only moderate dementia. This paper can be attacked on a number of grounds, such as possible biases in the choice of cases and the lack of objective psychological assessments, but at best it can only demonstrate that there is not a perfect correlation between intellectual changes and neuropathology.

By far the best investigation, and the one giving the most encouraging results, comes from the Newcastle group (Blessed et al., 1968; Roth et al., 1966 and 1967). There were 60 subjects in all. Of these 26 had dementia and the rest were normal elderly subjects, or elderly subjects with functional psychiatric disorders or who had had delirious states. Each patient was scored on a 28-point scale to measure the degree of dementia. Simple tests of orientation, recent and remote memory, and concentration were also administered. The brains were studied after autopsy and the neuropathological feature considered was the intensity of plaque formation. Over the whole group there was a highly significant correlation between the score on the dementia scale and the plaque count ($r = 0.77$). The inverse correlation between the plaque count and performance on the tests was also substantial ($r = 0.59$). As might be expected from the composition of the total group (including normal subjects and those with functional psychiatric disorders) there was an appreciable cluster of subjects with low plaque counts and good scores on the other variables. When these were eliminated the correlations between plaque count and the other variables fell to 0.64 for the dementia score and -0.52 for performance on the other tests. Nevertheless these correlations are still quite good and both are highly significant ($P < 0.001$).

The work of Roth and his associates is by far the most credible in this area. Their investigation uses larger numbers and is much better designed and described than those of Rothschild. From the published descriptions, the sceptic could set out to repeat the Newcastle study with some degree of accuracy. Rothschild's (1937 and 1942) papers do not meet this criterion. For these reasons much greater weight must be attached to the impressive correlations obtained by Roth and his associates than to Rothschild's negative evidence.

CEREBRAL BLOOD FLOW AND OXYGEN UPTAKE

It is well established that regional cerebral blood flow and oxygen uptake in the brain, as measured by such techniques as the xenon inhalation method, are reduced in patients with dementia (see the discussions of Simard *et al.*, 1971 and Oleson, 1974). There are a few reports of attempts to relate these physiological variables to psychological changes and some of these are somewhat deficient in terms of poor methodology and the small number of subjects used.

Lassen *et al.* (1957) had 19 middle-aged subjects, six of whom were normal and the rest were either likely or confirmed cases of dementia. Cerebral oxygen consumption was reduced in the demented subjects and the five subjects with the lowest oxygen uptake were all found to have strong evidence of cerebral atrophy on the AEG. Psychological functioning was assessed by a measure of fluctuation in digit learning and an adaptation of Weschsler's Block Design subtest. The authors claimed a rough relationship between oxygen uptake and psychological performance but no statistical details were given. On the basis of the small number of subjects and the rather arbitrary and inadequate psychological assessment it is doubtful if a significant correlation could have been achieved. Klee (1964) reported 11 new cases studied in a similar way who showed very similar results to those of Lassen *et al.* (1957).

In a later investigation, Lassen *et al.* (1960) determined cerebral oxygen uptake in eleven young normal adults, five elderly normal subjects and nine elderly demented patients. As might be expected the elderly normal subjects had lower uptake levels than the young normals, with those of the elderly demented patients being markedly depressed even by comparison with normal controls of a similar age. The psychological assessments were very much better than those used in Lassen's previous study and involved a psychiatric interview, administration of the Wechsler Adult Intelligence Scale, Raven's Progressive Matrices, the Bender Motor Gestalt, and other tests. A number of significant correlations were found between oxygen uptake and the various psychological measures but this was with data from both normal and abnormal groups combined.

In an earlier investigation, Lovett-Doust *et al.* (1953) administered most of the Wechsler–Bellevue Intelligence Scale subtests to 89 elderly subjects whose clinical conditions were alleged to represent a wide continuum of the effects of dementia and for whom arterial oxygen saturation had been assessed. A few subjects were lost in the calculation of the correlation coefficients because they were unable to complete the intelligence testing. The correlation between the physiological variable and IQ was found to be 0·56 for 77 subjects. The level of arterial oxygen saturation also had a significant correlation with the Tooting Bec Questionnaire which consists of a wide variety of questions dealing with simple items of information (both personal and non-personal) and with orientation.

Using the intra-arterial xenon injection technique it is possible to measure regional cerebral blood flow in different parts of the brain. Gustafson and Risberg (1974) used this technique with 50 cases of presenile dementia looking at eight regions of the dominant hemisphere. Symptoms of marked mental deterioration like amnesia, apraxia and aphasia, appeared to be particularly associated with reduced oxygen metabolism in the posterior temporal and occipito-parietal regions. Studies of this type in which psychological findings can be correlated with changes in particular parts of the brain are of considerable interest and it is to be hoped that further experiments of this type will be carried out.

THE ELECTROENCEPHALOGRAM AND OTHER NEUROPHYSIOLOGICAL VARIABLES

The general changes to be found in the electroencephalogram's (EEG) of demented subjects were outlined in Chapter Five. It has only been possible to trace one investigation that has directly related EEG variables to psychological changes and that is Short et al. (1968). They used 28 elderly female demented patients who were rated for both cognitive ability and emotional response (lability of affect, facial expression and warmth of response). Scores from the EEG were based on the percentage of alpha within the record and a global assessment of the abnormality of the EEG. The relationship between the EEG and the two psychological variables seemed to be curvilinear and so the correlation ratio was computed. This was statistically significant for both cognitive ability and emotional response.

Two other studies are possibly worth noting in this context. Müller and Grad (1974) found highly significant correlations between slowing of the EEG and both intellectual tests and psychiatric ratings of the clinical features of dementia. Unfortunately the sample of subjects used included the whole range of psychiatric disorders in the elderly as well as normal controls and only approximately 15% had dementia. In the other study, Wang et al. (1970) demonstrated a significant relationship between slowing of the EEG and the verbal-performance discrepancy on the Wechsler Adult Intelligence Scale using normal elderly subjects.

Speed of conduction in peripheral nerves has also been related to behavioural measures (Levy et al., 1970; Levy and Poole, 1966; see also Levy, 1972). Levy and Poole (1966) showed that peripheral nerve conduction is slower in demented elderly subjects than in non-demented subjects of a similar age. This finding was followed up by Levy et al. (1970) who found that conduction was allowed only in motor nerves and not in sensory nerves. The 47 subjects in their sample were also subjected to an independent psychiatric evaluation resulting in a rating of the degree of dementia and some psychological tests which were mainly concerned with memory. Significant correlations were found between motor nerve conduction velocity and both the ratings of dementia and a number of the specific psychological tests.

MORTALITY

Sanderson and Inglis (1961) gave the learning tests described by Walton and Black (1957) and Inglis (1959b) to two groups of elderly subjects. In the general style of Inglis' research, one of these groups was judged to be memory disordered (i.e., almost certainly demented) on clinical grounds and the other was thought to have no memory disorder. Survival at 16 months after testing was then related to both the clinical judgements of memory disorder and the memory tests. Clinical judgement was not significantly related to mortality despite the importance of a clinical impression of memory disorder in the diagnosis of dementia and Roth's (1955) demonstration of an association between dementia and early mortality. However, mortality had an appreciable correlation with the scores on the learning tests.

The ability of psychological tests to predict survival has been confirmed by other investigations. Hall *et al.* (1972) reported on the survival of subjects used in an early survey of the elderly. Decline in intelligence as judged from administration of the Wechsler Adult Intelligence Scale was found to predict death in both schizophrenics and dements, whilst a verbal learning impairment was associated with a failure to survive in the demented group only.

Probably the most convincing study in terms of its methodology is that of Jarvik and Falek (1963). Unfortunately their subjects were ordinary elderly individuals and not specially selected on the grounds of having dementia. These subjects were tested and retested on various subtests from the Wechsler and Stanford–Binet intelligence scales over a period of several years. The amount of decline in test performance was then related to survival 5 years after the last testing. It was found that those subjects who had what the authors describe as a 'critical' loss in test score had a much higher mortality.

MISCELLANEOUS FINDINGS

Of the few investigations that fall into this section two are biochemical. Gottfries *et al.* (1970) found a significant negative correlation between the levels of homovanillic acid in the cerebrospinal fluid of patients with senile dementia and ratings of intellectual deterioration, disturbance in social functioning and degree of emotional change. Similar correlations, although not always significant, were found in a much smaller group of subjects with presenile dementia. In the other biochemical investigation, Cox and Orme (1973) showed that serum levels of sodium and potassium were associated with scores on a dementia scale. This scale was based on the recall of information relating to dates, names and places.

The final reports concern the estimation of vibratory and other senses in elderly subjects. Whanger and Wang (1974) obtained a significant relationship between dementia and vibratory threshold which was measured at the wrist. It is unfortunate that the group on which the relationship was established contained both demented and normal subjects. It is possible that the correlation would be attenuated or might ever disappear if only demented subjects had been used. This paper does raise the possibility that some of the decline in functioning in demented patients might be related to sensory deficits. This possibility has been examined more closely by O'Neil and Calhoun (1975) who used measures relating to sensory efficiency in the auditory, visual and tactile modalities and related these to ratings and other simple assessments of behaviour. In general, the correlations were positive and significant. This finding has important implications for both research and clinical management and the role of sensory deficits in psychological dysfunction in demented subjects needs to be studied more closely.

COMMENT

Significant correlations between a wide range of nonpsychological variables (psychological, radiological, pathological, etc.) and various behavioural measures have been established well enough for there to be no real doubt that the psychological manifestations of dementia are related to the other changes that are alleged to occur. These correlations suggest that the different types of change are all produced by the same disease process. In order finally to prove this point of the unitary nature of dementia, it would be necessary to carry out multivariate analyses on data of all types taken from the same subject population. As yet no data suitable for this all-embracing type of analysis have been obtained.

Of course, not all the looked for correlations were found and some of those that emerged as statistically significant were often small in that they would account for only a small proportion of the total variance. As was argued at the beginning of this chapter, this situation is only to be expected because of the methodological problems involved and it is even surprising that some of the investigations were able to get the positive results that they did.

Taken as a whole the findings have two main implications of which the first is practical and the second theoretical. The low level of most of the correlations involved means that the level of one type of variable cannot be used to predict that of another. If all the varied manifestations claimed to be part of dementia are agreed to be the consequence of the same disease process, another implication of the low correlations is that dementia cannot be diagnosed accurately solely on the basis of an appropriate indication from one type of variable. The diagnosis can only be considered reliable when it is indicated by information gained from a number of different spheres.

Although there are probably few who would agree with them, there are a small number of writers on the subject of dementia who either deny a physcial basis or, whilst acknowledging the physical manifestations, consider these as irrelevant to the psychological features. Such theories will be examined in the next chapter, but for the present it is sufficient to note that the finding of correlations such as those described above makes any theoretical speculations on causation in which the physical changes do not hold a central place highly improbable.

Part Three
Implications for Theory and Practice

7
Psychology and Explanations of Dementia

Much of the psychological research into dementia is empirical in nature and few authors have concerned themselves with theoretical issues. This may well be partly be due to a feeling that, since dementia appears to be a disease process with causes that are not psychological, psychological research will not be relevant to explanatory models of dementia. The psychological work on dementia that has involved the most theoretical discussion has been that on memory and intellectual functioning, but even here the theoretical models have been those derived from the study of normal psychological functioning.

The question of what constitutes an adequate explanation of any phenomenon is extremely complex and the nature of the different types of explanation is a matter for philosophical discussion (e.g., White, 1967). It seems that there are two different types of explanation of relevance here. The first is a causal explanation in which the phenomenon under discussion is assumed to have been directly caused or produced by some other event or process. There can be little doubt that most psychological research on dementia implicitly assumes that a satisfactory causal explanation, when one is found, will be in terms of organic pathological processes.

The second type of explanation is in terms of laws. A law specifies certain relationships between variables without attempting to state what *caused* the circumstances to be such that the postulated relatiohsip holds good. A well known example of a law comes from elementary physics in the shape of Ohm's Law. This describes the relationship that holds between current, voltage and resistance in a simple direct current electrical circuit. Whilst it provides a very satisfactory explanation or prediction of how one of the triad of variables will behave when the others are altered, it says nothing at all about why the relationship came to be so. Most explanations in the physical sciences are laws and not cause and effect explanations and the achievements of physics indicate that laws can be extremely powerful and useful explanations.

With this in mind, psychological findings are relevant in three types of explanatory endeavour in dementia. The first is in the rare situations in which psychological factors have been assumed to be causal. Secondly, there are psychological explanations in the form of laws which aim to specify the relationships between psychological variables in dementia without any prejudice as to what caused the situation. Finally, some non-psychological theories do have psychological implications and the extent to which these are borne out by empirical evidence can be ascertained. This chapter is intended to deal with these three aspects and deliberately excludes the highly important non-psychological theories of dementia where psychological evidence is irrelevant.

THEORIES IN WHICH PSYCHOLOGICAL FACTORS HAVE BEEN CONSIDERED CAUSAL

There are very few theorists who have suggested that psychological factors are the major cause of dementia. One of these is Morgan (1965) who described the features of 'senility' and especially senile dementia as being a 'senescent defence against a personal and inevitable death'. The indication for this claim is that the memory disurbance in dementia is most apparent for recently experienced information. The patient's most recent memories would remind him of his age, increasing infirmity, and impending demise. Forgetting these things, argues Morgan, is the appropriate defence mechanism. It follows from this analysis that the appropriate therapeutic response to dementia is to institute psychotherapy aimed at reducing the patient's terror of death.

Morgan's theory is open to a number of severe criticisms. It can be ruled out as a total explanation of dementia in that it only attempts to account for the memory loss in dementia and has nothing to say about the large number of other changes, both psychological and non-psychological, that occur in dementia. As Caird (1966) has claimed, the theory in the form put forward by Morgan (1965) does not even satisfactorily cope with the memory disorder. There is experimental evidence that under many conditions the demented subject fails to acquire new information with normal facility, whereas Morgan implies that the information reaches memory storage with normal facility but is then repressed. Although Miller's (1975) experiment shows that, under certain circumstances, acquisition may be up to normal levels, this cannot be claimed as supporting evidence because Morgan's notion of repression would have difficulty in showing why a partial information condition could lead to normal levels of recall.

Morgan (1967) has defended his theory against Caird (1966) by arguing that the important question does not lie in the specific nature of the memory disturbance but in why it occurs at all. Regardless of how the process of repression is carried out, Morgan puts forward a specific prediction to show that repression is in operation. Using a normal type of memory experiment with words as the stimuli to be remembered, words relating to death would give a larger GSR response at the time of presentation in demented subjects and would also be more difficult to recall than neutral words. Morgan suggests that a test of his theory along these lines would be a simple matter. This is not so because of the need to match both neutral and death-related words for such characteristics as frequency of usage and for their ability to create emotional arousal in normal subjects. Death-related words could be emotionally arousing even for young subjects for whom death was not such an iminent threat, and a word's power to arouse emotion could be related to the ease with which it is remembered.

These methodological complications do not present an insuperable obstacle to the design of an adequate experiment but as yet no one appears to have considered it worthwhile to exploit this line of investigation. Possibly it is significant that Morgan himself has not published any further work on this subject.

Another theory in psychological terms is that of Rothschild (1937, 1942) and Rothschild and Sharp (1941). As we saw in the preceding chapter, Rothschild tried to relate psychological changes in dementia with the pathological findings at autopsy (loss of cells, number of plaques, etc.). In two separate investigations he failed to establish any relationship between pathological features and mental state. Rothschild then argued that, since the neuropathological features of dementia found in his studies were also identical with those found in normal ageing, dementia could not possibly be a direct consequence of these neuropathological changes to which it is not related and which are merely the features of a normal ageing process. He also advanced the opinion that there are a number of predisposed individuals who do not have the capacity to adapt to the usual neuropathological changes associated with ageing and therefore become demented.

Rothschild's basic premise is that the psychological and neuropathological features of dementia are unrelated. In the preceding chapter the evidence of relevance to this issue was discussed in some detail and it was concluded that there could be very little doubt that the organic changes in dementia are related to the mental features. It was also argued that there were potent methodological reasons why only the most carefully executed investigations would be likely to show significant correlations and Rothschild's studies were undoubtedly deficient in their design.

Although this theory must be rejected as it stands, Rothschild does raise the intriguing possibility that some individuals may be predisposed to develop dementia and that this predisposition may be related to psychological factors. Appropriate evidence is sparse but it has been suggested that dements have a characteristic premorbid personality which is of a rigid and obsessional nature (Noyes and Kolb, 1958). Oakley (1965) attempted to get empirical proof of this by interviewing the close relatives of a large number of female patients with senile dementia. The relatives were asked about the subjects' premorbid behaviour in terms of a number of questions derived from descriptions of the obsessional personality given in standard psychiatric textbooks. These questions were shown to have at least a minimal validity in measuring obsessionality in that a small group of diagnosed obsessionals showed a large number of the behavioural features covered by the questions.

As compared with non-demented control groups, the relatives of the demented patients certainly did report a higher incidence of obsessional characteristics. Nevertheless there are some problems which preclude accepting this result at face value. As Oakley is aware senile dementia has a very insidious onset and this makes it extremely difficult for relatives to know where the premorbid period ends. It is possible that when the first mild changes of dementia begin to appear the patient may well compensate to some extent by becoming more rigid and stereotyped in his behaviour. Especially when viewed in retrospect this might be easily confused with the characteristics of an obsessional personality.

Other evidence that psychological factors have any appreciable causal significance in dementia is hard to find. One exception is the retrospective study of 25 elderly female demented patients and a similar number of normal elderly subjects carried out by Amster and Krauss (1974). These authors attempt to identify 'life crises' occurring in the previous 5 years of their subjects' lives and discovered that the incidence of these was about double in the demented group. Amster and Krauss correctly point out that the causal direction is not established by this study but do not favour an interpretation that a developing dementing illness may in itself bring about more crisis situations. Another possibility, ignored by Amster and Krauss, is that once the dementing illness has started to get under way, the patient becomes less and less able to cope with the inevitable stresses and strains in normal life. These may then be elevated to the level of a major crisis in the demented individual's life. Amster and Krauss also link their findings with Wilson's psychosomatic approach to dementia. This is described more fully below but Wilson believes that the restricted view of life taken by some elderly persons leads to a restricted cerebral blood flow and hence dementia.

Social factors have also been implicated in the causation of dementia. For example, Williams *et al.* (1942) looked at the circumstances surrounding admission in groups of patients with senile and arteriosclerotic dementia. As compared with the arteriosclerotic group, those with senile dementia were less likely to have had financial security and were especially prone to loss of 'social integration' (i.e., not being a member of a close family group). Against this must be set the much more extensive and better executed epidemiological investigations of the Newcastle group (Garside *et al.*, 1965) which failed to find any evidence of direct social causation. It is possible that the conflict of evidence here lies in distinguishing between the causes of dementia and the factors that lead to hospitalization once the dementing process has started. The method used by Williams *et al.* (1942) would be likely to confound this distinction.

Theorists influenced by psychoanalysis have also tried to impute psychological factors in the aetiology of dementia. Ferenczi (1922) has developed the notion that injury to, or disease of, an organ results in the withdrawal of libido from ego functions in the outer world and focuses it on the affected area. This concentration on the self may evoke a return to an infantile state of narcissism. Taking as his example general paresis, Ferenczi argued that this transfer of the libido invests the brain with the qualities of an erogenous zone thus producing most of the varied psychological symptoms seen in general paresis. Only the 'neuraesthenic' symptoms of this disease are allowed to be the direct result of the organic process. Although Ferenczi developed this theoretical structure with the highly variable clinical features of general paresis in mind, there is little doubt that he would have extended this argument to postulate similar psychodynamic processes in other organic diseases of the brain as is implied by Brosin (1952). The approach certainly holds equal validity when applied to dementia.

At the very least this theory is very speculative and it must be emphasized that there is no experimental evidence that can be used in its support. Like many psychoanalytical formulations it is difficult to conceive of any unequivocal test that might be made. Possibly the most useful thing that can be derived from it is the general notion that some of the signs and symptoms of dementia might be caused primarily by the disease process whilst others could be the consequence of the patient's reaction to these basic changes. It is conceivable that, at least in some cases, depression could result from the patient's reaction to the experience of finding that some of his powers are fading. Other possibilities could be suggested but this general idea has not yet been given any serious consideration by investigators.

The remaining attempt to handle dementia in terms of causal psychological mechanisms is to see the condition as a psychosomatic disease. Wilson (1955) allows that pathological changes within the brain may well be the direct cause of the symptoms seen in dementia but claims that these pathological changes may in turn be the result of psychological factors. He postulates that the older individual's life may become narrow and meaningless. The inevitably restricted view of life then leads to a restricted blood flow. This subsequently leads to the observed pathological and psychological features of dementia. Needless to say this is the psychosomatic approach at its most naive. The nature of the mechanism which could link a restricted life style with a restricted blood flow is unspecified and to claim that restriction of one thing claims to restriction in the other surely descends to the level of argument by 'clang association'. Wilson offers no real evidence in favour of his speculations and none has been published since.

In summary, the only firm conclusion that emerges from examining theories which claim that psychological factors are causal in dementia, is that none of them poses any serious threat to the predominant view that the basic cause is organic. It is still possible that psychological mechanisms could play a contributory role in aetiology but this has yet to be convincingly proved. By far the most likely possibility is that some of the features associated with dementia, especially in its early stages, may be the result of the patient's reaction to his decreasing capacities.

NON-CAUSAL PSYCHOLOGICAL THEORIES

As has been described above we can have valid and useful theories which are not causal in nature. These specify laws or relationships without attempting to describe how that particular situation happened to arise in the first place. To some degree we have already encountered this type of explanation in trying to describe the varied features of memory disorder in dementia in terms of short-term or long-term memory stores, or in claiming that the intellectual changes can all be subsumed under the general principle of a loss of the abstract attitude. These deal only with one aspect of the symptomatology of dementia and this section will examine theories which could be used to explain a wide range of symptoms as being manifestations of a disturbance in a single, more fundamental, process.

A common approach for this type of explanation has been to fall back on the concept of arousal or one of its related notions. Post (1966) has suggested that demented patients have a lowered level of cerebral excitation and this might explain their poor memory. Although not quite so explicitly brought out by Post, lowered cerebral excitation could be used to explain all the cognitive changes in dementia and some of the non-cognitive features as well.

Hemsi *et al.* (1968) attempted a direct test of this hypothesis using a group of elderly dements and a group of elderly depressives matched for age. Their indices of arousal were sleep thresholds and the level of unstimulated salivation. According to the theory the depressed group might have some lowering of arousal but this would not be as great as that occurring in the dements. In line with expectations the demented group had lower sleep thresholds, but the measures of unstimulated salivation implied a lower level of arousal in the depressed group. The demented group also performed less well on a range of psychometric tests including tests of intelligence and memory. It is difficult to draw any firm conclusions from this experiment. Arousal is a difficult thing to measure and it is well established that the various psychophysiological parameters commonly used in attempts to quantify the concept of arousal do not always agree (Duffy, 1962). As the authors point out, arousal may not be a unitary variable but they emphasize the heuristic value of theories based on arousal.

A more complicated thesis involving arousal has been put forward by Kendrick (1972). Kendrick bases his ideas on Routtenberg's (1968) theoretical discussion of arousal in which he postulates two arousal systems. The first of these (AS1) is based on the reticular activating system whilst the second arousal system (AS2) is a function of activity within the limbic system. Routtenberg views these two systems as being mutually inhibitory with AS1 being related to 'drive' and AS2 to 'incentive'. A high level of AS1 maintains incoming stimuli and the activation of AS2 after any incoming information will allow that information to be consolidated into other than temporary storage. Because AS2 supresses AS1, this prevents fresh incoming stimuli from interfering with the consolidation process. According to Kendrick, AS1 is involved in short-term memory whilst AS2 fulfils the underlying physiological component of 'reinforcement'.

Kendrick (1972) extends this by hypothesizing that the lowered cortical excitation occurring in dementia is mediated by irreversible changes which have occurred in both of Routtenberg's arousal systems. He also suggests that depression can sometimes produce changes in AS2. This latter proposition is needed to explain why some depressed patients perform as badly as many dements on learning tests like Kendrick's Synonym Learning Test (learning and other tests used in the diagnosis of dementia will be described in Chapter

Eight). This is assumed to be because learning tests require both AS1 and AS2 activity. Kendrick alleges that his Digit Copying Test will reflect the level of AS1 only and scores on this test should be poor in demented but not in depressed patients. He then goes on to re- analyse data presented in previous publications in an attempt to confirm predictions from this theory.

On the whole the theory comes out quite well in terms of fitting in with the appropriate predictions, but two reservations must be entered. Firstly, Kendrick's version of the low arousal hypothesis was inspired to a considerable degree by problems arising from data obtained with his Synonym Learning and Digit Copying tests, especially the occasional inability of these tests to discriminate between patients with dementia and those with depression. It is hardly surprising that when substantially this same data is re-analysed, it should fit the new theory. As yet we do not know if Kendrick is taking the essential further step of making fresh predictions and testing these out by the collection of new data. The second reservation applies to Kendrick's whole style of theorizing. He starts from the specific neurophysiological function of a small part of the brain, e.g. the reticular activating system, and proposes to measure this by means of psychological tests without any real evidence of a link between the two. It is a far cry from the specific neuronal activity of a small unit of the brain to the speed with which a subject can copy rows of digits. The whole history of work on arousal shows that its measurement is no simple matter and great reservation must be expressed regarding its equation with a single behavioural index.

A hypothesis which could readily be related to that of low arousal is expressed by Bower (1967). Bower acknowledges that the basic aetiology of senile dementia is organic. However, the organic changes reduce the functional capacity of the individual and this results in lower environmental demands being placed upon him. The position then is that the afflicted person suffers a mild form of sensory deprivation. Sensory deprivation, which is known to have marked effects on young adults, can then be used to explain some of the psychological features of dementia. Bower offers some evidence that enriched environmental experience for patients with senile dementia does result in improvements as would be predicted from this theory (see also Chapter Nine for further evidence on this point).

The construction of a good psychological model of dementia is a theoretical exercise that has yet to be undertaken. Arousal could still prove to be a useful concept in this model although it suffers from a severe handicap in the hands of many psychologists who introduce it by many devious and almost untestable means to explain well nigh anything. A sound psychological model of dementia would be of tremendous value in any efforts that might be made to ameliorate the consequences of dementia.

NON-PSYCHOLOGICAL THEORIES WITH PSYCHOLOGICAL IMPLICATIONS

It is far beyond the scope of this book (and of its author) to argue the merits or demerits of any non-psychological explanations of dementia in the terms in which they were originally proposed. Nevertheless such theories can have important psychological implications and these will now become the focus of attention.

A common explanation of dementia is that it represents an abnormally rapid ageing of the nervous system (Brain and Walton, 1969; Critchley, 1933; Miller, 1974c). In many ways this is an attractive hypothesis with much to support it when considered at a superficial level. The brain loses cells and shows some ventricular dilatation in normal ageing. Most of the recorded neuropathological changes in dementia are also found to a lesser degree in the brains of neurologically normal elderly subjects, although some neuropathologists have doubted if the neuropathological features of normal ageing and Alzheimer's disease are absolutely identical (Bender *et al.*, 1970; Dayan, 1971). The EEG changes in dementia have also been described as an exaggeration of the effects of normal ageing. This list of similarities could be extended considerably and it cannot be denied that the whole picture in dementia has much in common with what could be imagined as the effects of normal ageing of the nervous system writ large. The crucial question is not whether the two processes are similar, which they undoubtedly are, but whether they can be considered to be absolutely identical. This is of more than academic interest because it affects the search for the basic cause of dementia in that this could lie within the mechanisms responsible for ageing, or the condition could be produced by an independent disease process which compounds and distorts the effects of normal ageing.

Since the brain is the organ responsible for the control of behaviour, it follows that if the accelerated ageing hypothesis is correct then the behavioural effects of dementia should match those of normal ageing. There is a fair amount of evidence that might be considered to have a bearing on this point but it will be argued later that answering this question is not as simple as it might seem at first sight.

As far as performance on intelligence tests is concerned the effects of normal ageing are well documented (see Chapter 2 and Savage, 1973), and something is also known about the consequences of dementia. There are a number of similarities in the two patterns of decline. On the Wechsler intelligence scales, patients with dementia usually have lower IQs on the performance scale than on the verbal scale (see Chapter 3). A similar general tendency to show a more rapid decline on the subtests of the performance scale in normal ageing can be deduced from the stadardization data given in Wechsler's (1955) manual for the Wechsler Adult Intelligence Scale. Despite this, the patterns of change on the individual Wechsler subtests may still not be identical. Botwinnick and Birren (1951b) specifically examined this point and found that the subtests showing the greatest decline in raw scores as a result of normal ageing were not those that gave maximum discrimination between demented and non-demented old people. Dorken and Greenbloom (1953) similarly concluded that the pattern of subtest changes in dementia is different. On the other hand, Rabin's (1945) data reveals no change in the pattern of subtest changes for demented subjects, and Whitehead (1973b) also concluded that the pattern of subtest scores in dementia was no different from that occurring in a group of depressed patients of a similar age. (It is assumed that the effect of depression on intelligence-test scores is negligible.)

Some other investigators using psychometric tests have also failed to support the accelerated ageing hypothesis. Dorken and Kral (1951) in their study based on the Rorschach technique concluded that the features shown by demented patients were not simply an exaggeration of those obtained in normal ageing. This same conclusion was endorsed by Dorken (1954) in his detailed review of a number of psychometric investigations carried out on demented patients.

Turning from psychometric to experimental investigations again reveals a certain amount of evidence that is not consistent with the accelerated-ageing hypothesis. The work on memory reviewed in Chapter Four gives a number of examples. Kral's argument for two distinct types of memory disorder is difficult to reconcile with the hypothesis, as is the work of Inglis and his associates on dichotic listening which showed the demented subjects to have a selective loss of information presented to the ear that was reported second. The accelerated-ageing hypothesis would lead to the prediction that the dements should be impaired relative to the elderly controls on both ears. Miller's (1975) demonstration that dements, but not age-matched controls, benefit from the presence of partial information at recall is also indicative of processes occurring in the demented subject that are not manifest in the normal.

Straumanis et al. (1965) examined visually evoked responses on the EEG and compared elderly demented subjects with age-matched normal controls and also with a group of younger normal subjects. The effects of normal ageing were found to be particularly marked on the components of the response occurring within the first 100 milliseconds. The dements differed from the normal controls of similar age in the components manifest after the first 100 milliseconds. This experiment is one of the most difficult to reconcile with the accelerated-ageing hypothesis. In a study of the verbal transformation effect, Obusek and Warren (1973) also compared the effects of dementia with those of normal ageing. The effect of normal ageing had previously been established as a lowering of both the number of verbal transformation effects and of the number of phonemic changes within those effects. Dements were found to differ from the normal aged in having an even lower number of transformation effects. So far this is consistent with the hypothesis under examination, but what is not is the finding that dements have a greater number of phonemic changes in those transformations that did occur. On this latter variable the dements were comparable to normal 10-year-old children.

The effect of normal ageing on motor skills has received some attention (e.g., Singleton, 1954; Welford, 1962). It is generally agreed that the retardation in motor performance that accompanies normal ageing is a consequence of slower decision processes in determining when and how to move rather than a slower speed of movement per se. In Miller's (1974a) experiment on motor speed in dementia it was found that whilst decision times were longer in the demented group, the biggest difference lay in the speed of execution of the movements.

The immediately preceding paragraphs give just some of the evidence pertinent to the issue under discussion. It could be argued in defence of the accelerated-ageing hypothesis, and with some justification, that the findings described were just a small proportion of those that might have been included, and furthermore that they were a sample very heavily biased towards those investigations that might be considered inconsistent with the hypothesis. The other side of the coin is that the accelerated-ageing hypothesis postulates identity between the consequences of ageing and dementia, with the sole exception of the rate at which they occur, and all that is required to refute the hypothesis is a single, well established, inconsistency.

Despite the appreciable amount of evidence that is apparently against it, the accelerated-ageing hypothesis is far from dead. This is because serious methodological criticisms can be advanced against all previous tests of the hypothesis (or, more correctly, experiments later presumed to be possible tests of the hypothesis since many of those cited were not originally designed with this question in mind). The methodological complications never seem to have been satisfactorily articulated until recently (Miller, 1974c). As a result of this, the evidence presented above can, at the very best, only be considered as suggestive. Because this theory of dementia is important it is worthwhile digressing on to the topic of what might constitute an adequate test of the theory.

The whole problem is reminiscent of the discussions surrounding the question of matching for mental age in experimental work with mentally handicapped children. (e.g., Baumeister, 1967; Clarke and Clarke, 1973). The crucial point is that the accelerated-ageing hypothesis predicts that the demented subject of a given age will give results on any relevant measure (and this is not restricted to psychological variables) identical with those of an older normal subject. In consequence the appropriate normal control group does not consist of normal subjects of the same age but of older normal subjects whose brains have advanced to the same degree of atrophy, plaque formation, etc. as the brains of the demented group. Such a control group has never been used and would be well nigh impossible to establish in any direct way.

The demented subject is usually compared with normal subjects of a similar age and the comparison is examined in the light of changes as a result of normal ageing up to the age of the demented group. This is not specifically indicated as being the case in many reports, which often do not include data dealing with the effect of normal ageing but merely refer to appropriate information obtained from other studies. However this is what it amounts to in practice. The experiment of Straumanis et al. (1965) on visually evoked responses is one of the most sophisticated in that it does contain a younger control group to establish the pattern of normal ageing up to the age of the two older groups. This experiment, in common with all the others, is open to the objection that, for a variety of reasons, the pattern in measures of normal age change may not be consistent over time. Specifically the normal changes occurring after the age of the demented group may not show the same pattern as those which appear before that age (e.g., age changes may be manifest at first during the first 100 milliseconds of the evoked response but after a certain age, later portions of the response may be more affected). As a result it is still possible that any differences between the demented and the age-matched normal control subjects could reflect the effects of a more advanced normal ageing.

Although simple in principle, this methodological complication is difficult to deal with in practical terms. The demented subject does not come ready labelled with an age that might correspond to the level of deterioration in his brain and there is no ethically justifiable way of matching subjects for neuropathological features. One solution to this difficulty was suggested by Miller (1974c). Demented subjects could be matched with older normal subjects on one variable known to be subject to appreciable change with age and then the two groups could be compared using other variables. For example, Miller's (1974a) experiment on motor skills could be re-designed to test the accelerated-ageing hypothesis by matching the group with presenile dementia with an older group of normal subjects on the basis of their speed of decision making. The two groups could then be compared on the time taken to execute the movements. A difference appearing under these circumstances would then give a less equivocal refutation of the accelerated-ageing hypothesis. Even this would not result in an ideal experiment because the older control group would have had different life experiences from the younger demented group (e.g., having been retired for longer). Nevertheless it would give a much better control than any previous experiment.

Another hypothesis for which psychological evidence is of direct relevance is that put forward by Corsellis (1970). Corsellis has pointed out that the most marked pathological changes in Alzheimer's disease occur in the region of the hippocampus. Because bilateral damage to the hippocampi is known to produce profound memory disturbances in human subjects, as in the well known Montreal case HM (e.g., Milner, 1966), Corsellis argues that the hippocampal changes in Alzheimer's disease might underlie the memory disturbances in that condition.

There has only been one experiment, that of Miller (1973), which has looked at memory disturbances in Alzheimer's disease in a way that is comparable to other studies of patients with bilateral hippocampal lesions. This experiment gave evidence of impairments in both long- and short-term memory in Alzheimer's disease, whilst the investigation of bilateral hippocampal subjects using a similar technique found that only long-term memory was affected (Drachman and Arbit, 1965). There are also other failures to find short-term memory impairments in cases with bilateral hippocampal lesions (e.g., Wickelgren, 1968) but Chapter Four revealed extensive evidence of short-term memory defects in dementia.

The issue becomes more complicated if we follow the implicit assumption made by some researchers into amnesia (e.g., Warrington and Weiskrantz,

1970) that the nature of the amnesic disturbance found in bilateral hippocampal lesions is the same as that occurring in Korsakoff's syndrome. Miller (1975) obtained the same effects of cueing on the long-term recall of demented patients as did Warrington and Weiskrantz (1970), who used a mixed group of patients with severe amnesias containing both cases with bilateral hippocampal lesions and with Korsakoff's syndrome. There is also a difference of opinion between research groups in London (Warrington, Weiskrantz and their associates) and in Boston (Cermak, Butters and others, e.g., Cermak *et al.*, 1971) as to whether patients with these severe amnesic syndromes show short-term memory impairments. Butters and Cermak (1974) give some strong arguments in favour of their view that short-term memory deficits do exist.

The essential prediction from Corsellis (1970) that the memory disturbance in Alzheimer's disease would match that found in bilateral hippocampal lesions, does not gain any support from the one experiment that has attempted to replicate the results found in one type of subject with those found in the other. However the picture becomes much less clear if it is allowed that the type of amnesia in bilateral hippocampal lesions is similar to that found in Korsakoff's syndrome. The varied findings in these severe amnesias do not give a solid enough basis for an unequivocal comparison with findings in Alzheimer's disease.

As presented here, the non-psychological theories do not emerge too well in terms of their psychological implications. With regard to the very important accelerated-ageing hypothesis, the only sure conclusion must be that this has never been adequately tested in terms of an experiment that has achieved the best possible design and included an older normal control group. It is obvious that normal ageing processes must have some influence on the behaviour of demented subjects but the available evidence points to the likelihood that a simple accelerated ageing of the nervous system cannot account for everything (Miller, 1974c).

CLOSING COMMENTS

Dementia is not a topic that has aroused much theoretical interest. An acceptable causal explanation has yet to be evolved and when it appears it is most unlikely to be psychological in nature. It is even possible that such a theory, when it emerges, may not have any direct psychological implications and so lie outside the present area of concern.

What is very much needed, and what may also be of much more practical value, is a good psychological model of dementia (i.e., a non-causal model). Whilst the effective medical treatment of most cases of dementia remains impossible, the only therapeutic approach that is available is to manipulate environmental conditions in order to improve the demented patient's quality of life and minimize his impairments. Such action can be most effectively carried out when we have a sound model of how the demented subject functions. Such notions as a low arousal level in dementia do have some limited implications for management in that they imply that raising the general level of background stimulation may improve functioning (just how effective this appears to be can be seen in Chapter 9). Unfortunately derivations of this type are at a very low level of specificity and furthermore a large number of other possible models could also lead to the same implication.

8
The Psychological Assessment of the Patient with Possible Dementia

In the practical application of psychological principles and techniques to the solution of clinical problems arising from dementia there are two main issues. The first is that of identifying dementia when it occurs and evaluating its characteristics within the individual patient. The second is the amelioration of the effects of dementia so that the afflicted person can achieve the maximum quality of life over his remaining years. These two aspects can be conveniently referred to as assessment and management.

A strong case could be put forward to support the argument that psychology is likely to make its most valuable contribution in the area of management. The potential value of psychology in management has not been matched by an extensive research interest in the problems of management which have only become an active area of concern within the past few years. The question of management and amelioration will be taken up in the next chapter. The present concern is with assessment which, in contrast, has enjoyed considerable attention over a long period although it is probably fair to say that interest in assessment is on the decline.

The literature on psychological assessment that could be considered to have some possible relevance to dementia really is vast. It is also extremely tedious to work through, especially for those who lack a taste for the minutiae of psychometric investigations. Since a large part of the literature is of very poor quality or consists of minor permutations on the same basic themes, the reader's boredom can be relieved by confining present consideration to major trends within those approaches which have attempted to conform to the usually accepted guidelines for work on psychometric tests. It is extremely doubtful whether the limitations on the selection of material dealt with in this chapter will lead to any appreciable distortion in the conclusions that are drawn.

There are two overlapping points of interest in the psychological assessment of dementia. The first is the measurement of the amount of deterioration. In practice it is usually the extent of deterioration in general intellectual functioning that is looked at and not the amount of decline in other psychological functions. Many psychologists have tried to devise means of assessing the degree of intellectual change that has occurred in a demented patient as compared with the individual's premorbid level of functioning. As we shall see, the decline occurring after the patient has presented with the condition is typically all that can be measured with any degree of accuracy.

The second problem is that of differential diagnosis. The most important diagnostic discrimination involving demented patients for which psychometric assessment is relevant, is that between dementia and functional psychiatric disorders, especially depression. Older people may present to psychiatric clinics in a withdrawn, uncommunicative state, possibly physically neglected if they have been living alone, and with an apparently low affect. On purely clinical grounds it can be very difficult to decide whether this picture is the result of depression or dementia. Unlike many of the exercises in differential diagnosis in which clinical psychologists have been extensively involved, this one is of some practical consequence since it has important implications for both treatment and prognosis.

THE MEASUREMENT OF INTELLECTUAL DECLINE

The ideal way to measure intellectual decline would be to compare a patient's level of functioning on a given test with results obtained from the same test just prior to the onset of the illness. This is only very occasionally possible in practice because few people that are encountered as patients have had any psychometric assessments carried out previously. In the few instances in which a patient has been tested before the results may be unobtainable or of little value. There may be inadequate information about the circumstances under which the previous result was obtained (e.g., when the case notes just record an IQ figure from a long past admission with not even a mention of the test on which it is based). Alternatively the necessary information may be available but indicates that the result was not reliable enough to form a basis for future comparisons. Even if these obstacles are overcome and there is sound data from a well described previous occasion, the time at which this data was obtained is of great importance. Results obtained early in adult life may not be above suspicion because there is very little information as to how stable relative performance on intellectual tests remains throughout the span of adult life for normal individuals (published data on ageing nearly always describes group means which could hide very wide individual variations). A result obtained too near the presumed onset of a possible dementing illness may have been contaminated by the disease process thus lowering the allegedly premorbid assessment and making the occurrence of a marked decline less likely (the insidious onset of most dementing illnesses means that it is only possible to guess at the date of onset.)

Direct measurement of intellectual decline can be made relatively easily from the point at which the patient comes to the notice of the service. A test can be administered and then repeated, or a parallel form given, at some later date. In the case of demented subjects this second testing usually needs to be at least a few months later if any measurable decline is to be found. Because of the inevitable delay this procedure is normally only of value where the diagnosis remains in doubt. Repeated testing after the patient has first presented also cannot reveal the total extent of the deline from premorbid levels and it also requires the use of a test with high reliability.

In any direct measurement of intellectual decline a point which must be borne in mind, and which is sometimes neglected even by experienced psychologists, is that test scores can change solely as a result of administering the same test a second time. Partly this is due to errors of measurement (and hence the need to keep these at a minimum by using tests of high reliability) but partly also because a gain in score commonly occurs as a result of practice. Gains due to practice even occur when using parallel forms of the same test as with Forms I and II of the Wechsler Bellevue Scales (Gerboth, 1950). It is often not appreciated how large gains on re-testing can be and thus a subject who gets an IQ of, say, 92 at first testing and one of 94 on re-testing may be assumed to have shown no significant change. However, test–re-test gains of around 15 IQ points have been shown for some scales and if this is the case for the test used with our hypothetical patient, it places his gain of only 2 IQ points in quite a different light.

It is unfortunate that there is a very limited amount of information available on the test–re-test characteristics of most intellectual tests and this is especially so where older subjects are involved. This paucity of data is probably not only because test–re-test studies are extremely tedious to carry out but because their value is often not fully recognized. Some indication of the likely changes in normal people can be obtained from Gerboth (1950) and Hamister (1949) for the Wechsler–Bellevue Scales; from Guertin et al. (1962) and Matarazzo (1973) for the Wechsler Adult Intelligence Scale and from Desai (1952) for Raven's Progressive Matrices. The simple statistical procedures required to make use of this information to its maximum effect are described by Payne and Jones (1957).

The difficulties inherent in the direct assessment of intellectual decline have led to many attempts to develop indirect methods. Since most are based on the same basic principle and are open to the same criticisms, there is little point in dealing with them all individually. The discussion can most usefully be carried out in general terms with minimal details of particular tests or indices of decline. It should also be pointed out that these indirect techniques were often originally designed for the assessment of all kinds of 'brain damage' or even to measure the intellectual decline that might occur in functional psychoses. Present concern lies solely with their possible use with demented patients although many of the arguments are quite general and would apply irrespective of the patient populations with which the techniques might be used.

Indirect methods of estimating intellectual decline are usually based on the assumption that some aspects of intellectual functioning are very prone to disruption by neurological disease whilst others are resistant to change. One popular assumption is that scores on vocabulary tests remain very stable. Since vacabulary is considered to be a particularly good indicator of general intelligence, a vocabulary test can be used as an index of premorbid intelligence. Other tests considered to measure abilities rather more prone to deterioration can be used to measure present intellectual status. The difference between the two then gives the extent of any intellectual deterioration. Tests of mental deterioration based on this principle have enjoyed considerable popularity. The best known of these are the Babcock–Levy Revised Examination for the Efficiency of Mental Functioning, the Hunt Minnesota Test for Organic Brain Damage, and the Shipley–Hartford Retreat Scale.

The principles underlying the use of vocabulary as an index of premorbid intelligence have been most authoritatively reviewed by Yates (1956) whose paper still remains the best single reference on the topic. As Yates points out, a number of assumptions are involved, the most crucial of these being that vocabulary tests can provide a good enough prediction of the level of intelligence in normal subjects; that vocabulary is resistant to the deleterious effects of brain pathology, and that vocabulary remains reasonably stable with age. This last assumption is necessary because it is intended to use vocabulary level at one point in time to predict general intelligence some time previously, and therefore there should be no change in vocabulary purely as the result of the ageing process which has been operative during that period. This assumption appears to be substantially true throughout the major part of adult life although vocabulary probably does decline in extreme old age.

Important objections can be raised against the other two assumptions. With regard to the claim that vocabulary is a good enough predictor of general intelligence, there is no need to present a detailed account of the evidence as this has been most ably done by Yates (1956). In general the situation is that vocabulary scales do correlate highly with overall measures of general intelligence and more highly than most other scales measuring specific abilities, but the level of the correlation is not high enough to avoid an appreciable margin of error in estimating IQ on this basis alone. The Wechsler Adult Intelligence Scale is probably not atypical in this respect. The exact figures depend upon the age level selected but there is always a highly significant (in the statistical sense) correlation between the score on the vocabulary subtest and the full scale IQ of around 0·8 (Wechsler, 1955). The application of basic statistical principles relating to measurement shows that even with such a high correlation, the standard error of prediction when full scale IQ is predicted from vocabulary alone is of the order of 10 IQ points. A large drop in present IQ as assessed by other tests (which usually correlate less well with overall IQ) would have to occur before it could be considered significantly different from the IQ estimate based on vocabulary alone.

The stability of vocabulary during pathological changes to the brain is also open to dispute. There are reports which claim to have found no decline in vocabulary in patients with definite brain disease (e.g., Gonen and Brown, 1968). On the other hand, there are also many investigations which have found the contrary. Acklesberg (1944) showed that scores on vocabulary tests correlated with the degree of dementia in a series of patients with senile dementia. Nelson's (1953) patients with organic brain pathology were observed to have markedly depressed scores on the Binet vocabulary scale as compared to a group of matched normal controls. The table of mean Wechsler subtest scores (Table 4, p. 35) shows vocabulary to have the least decline on average when compared with the other subtests, but the mean for vocabulary is still below the expected mean of 10·0. Whilst, on balance, vocabulary does seem susceptible to decline there is some evidence (Yacorzynski, 1941; Yates, 1956) that the susceptibility of vocabulary tests to decline is related to the criteria used by the test in determining whether the subject knows the meaning of a word. As one might expect, the more severe the criteria the more sensitive the test to cerebral pathology.

Another important difficulty with this type of indirect measurement of intellectual deterioration arises from the fact that subjects in their premorbid state are not always equally good (or bad) at all types of intellectual test. It is quite often the case that people with fairly high academic achievements (e.g. those having university degrees) are better at verbally oriented tasks such as vocabulary scales than they are at the performance type of task. Since the former is used to estimate 'premorbid' intelligence and the latter to give 'present' intelligence, subjects like this have an inbuilt tendency to show 'intellectual decline' even before they start dementing. The reverse pattern of abilities can be found amongst other subgroups within the general population and these may therefore show no deterioration for some time after a real decline has started.

In general terms the assumptions underlying the use of vocabulary to measure premorbid intelligence are only very rough approximations of the real situation. The important practical question is whether they hold up well enough for scales like the Babcock–Levy to be used in the measure of intellectual decline in the individual patient. The answer here is definitely 'No'. This is confirmed by studies of the discriminative power of these tests which have compared groups of 'organic' subjects (who may be presumed to have suffered intellectual deterioration) and neurologically normal controls. Whilst the group means may differ in the expected direction, the degree of overlap between the groups is so large as to preclude the making of reliable decisions about any individual patient. This is the conclusion that is revealed by Yates' (1954) review of the then existing data and since that time no one appears to have published any data which would merit any serious reconsideration of that opinion.

Conceptually similar attempts to measure intellectual deterioration are provided by the various deterioration indices based on the Wechsler intelligence scales. These scales base their assessment of intelligence on the combined results of 10 or 11 subtests, and it is well established that scores on some subtests decline more rapidly than others as a result of normal ageing. The further assumption is made that the pattern of intellectual deterioration produced by organic brain disease will follow the same pattern as that produced by ageing. Wechsler (1958) suggested that comparison of the scores on the four subtests least susceptible to deterioration with scores on the four most likely to deteriorate would yield a deterioration index.

The two groups of subtests selected by Wechsler are designated as the 'hold' and 'don't hold' tests respectively. The suggested 'hold' tests for the Wechsler Adult intelligence Scale are Vocabulary, Information, Object Assembly and Picture Completion. The 'don't hold' tests are Digit Span, Similarities, Digit Symbol and Block Design (Wechsler, 1958). Others have been dissatisfied with Wechsler's deterioration index and have suggested their own indices based on different subtest groupings (e.g., Hewson, 1949; Reynell, 1944). Again there is little point in giving a detailed account of each of them because the arguments applied to one of these indices almost invariably hold for all the rest.

The criticisms that can be advanced against these indices generally mirror those that have already been sct out in evaluating the use of vocabulary in the measurement in intellectual decline. There is first of all the gratuitous assumption that the pattern of decline in subtest scores is exactly the same in normal ageing as it is in neurological disease. This assumption is flatly contradicted by the substantial literature which purports to show differential changes in Wechsler subtest scores across different types of brain damage (e.g., Meier and French, 1966). If there are different patterns of subtest changes produced by brain damage, then only one of these (if any) can match the pattern of change produced by normal ageing.

In effect the deterioration index is using a small group of subtests (usually only four) to estimate premorbid intelligence and another small group to indicate the present IQ level. Because of this they cannot have the reliability of the full test and the error of measurement will be increased. As a result, differences between the two estimates will have to be large to be considered outside the range of chance variation. Normal subjects will also tend to have an uneven pattern of performance on the subtests. Any individual may have been naturally better or worse on the 'hold' tests and so have an initial bias for or against showing deterioration.

By far the most important criticism of the use of deterioration indices comes from the many empirical studies which show that discrimination using this type of index is very poor. One recent example comes from Savage (1971) who presents data in which an 'organic' group and a normal group of elderly subjects are compared on the Wechsler Deterioration Index. Although the groups are well separated in terms of their mean scores on the index, there is considerable overlap in the distribution. This is to such as extent that about a quarter of the allegedly deteriorated organic group emerge as having less intellectual deterioration than the typical normal subject of the same age. This is again too low a level of accuracy for making meaningful decisions about the individual patient. For a few psychologists the search for the right Wechsler subtest combination still goes on, rather like the mediaeval alchemists search for the philosopher's stone, and with as little likelihood of ultimate success. Occasionally reports of new indices which seem to approach useful levels of discrimination do appear (e.g., Crookes, 1974) but these either lack the crucial confirmation by cross-validation or break down when attempts at cross-validation are made.

A final method of estimating deterioration is to use the patient's past history, especially his educational attainments and occupational status, as a guide to what his intellectual level must have been. It is fairly obvious that a patient with higher education and a successful professional career who gives a current IQ of 85 has suffered appreciable intellectual decline. Unfortunately cases as clear cut as this are rare and considerable difficulty arises because of the large variation in measured IQ found amongst subjects from the same occupational groups or with the same educational attainments. This is well illustrated by Harrell and Harrell's (1945) report of the measured IQs of various occupational groups entering the United States armed services during the Second World War. Even high status professional groups like lawyers, with a mean IQ well above the population mean, show considerable variation and the proportion who have IQs of around 100 is far from negligible. Unskilled workers may have an average IQ below the population mean of 100 but the range of variation is much wider than it is for professional groups. Unskilled labourers of rather better than average intelligence are not uncommon.

A similar pattern emerges in the case of educational attainments. High educational qualifications may guarantee a certain minimal level of intelligence but a very poor school record does not mean that the person could not have been highly intelligent. It can readily be seen that the measurement of deterioration using a patient's educational and occupational background as an indication of premorbid intelligence, is least reliable in the case of patients with low occupational status who opted out of the educational system at the earliest opportunity. It is just this type of patient who is encountered most frequently in practice.

Apart from the rare instance of the patient for whom there is reliable previous test data that is also accessible, there is no satisfactory way of measuring intellectual deterioration from the premorbid level. All that can be offered with accuracy is the measurement of any subsequent decline once the problem has come to notice. All the indirect methods are suspect but occasionally a patient will present with an educational level or occupational status which indicates that his IQ must once have been superior to that obtained at present testing. In such cases the intellectual deterioration may well be so obvious on clinical grounds that the psychiatrist or neurologist does not need to make a referral for psychological assessment.

There is a final, and more technical, qualification that must be entered with regard to any assessment of change in IQ. IQ is not an interval scale and, as a consequence, a fall in IQ of, say, 10 points cannot be assumed to represent the same degree of change in intellectual ability when occurring across different portions of the possible range of IQ. A direct corollary of this is that intelligence tests are likely to vary in their sensitivity to change depending upon what starting point the change is to be measured from.

DIAGNOSTIC TESTS

Diagnostic tests do not set out to measure a change but to distinguish between patients of two or more different types. Because clinical psychology has developed largely within a psychiatric setting, the available tests have often been devised to separate 'organic' states from functional psychiatric disorders. In practice the most important differential diagnosis for which these tests are relevant is that between dementia and depression. These two conditions can present with a very similar clinical picture in which the patient is unresponsive, neglected and with an apparently low affect. Unlike many of the differential diagnoses in psychiatry to which clinical psychologists have applied their efforts, this one does have important implications both for management and prognosis.

In line with most other parts of this chapter attention will be selective and focused only upon the most useful instruments in the differential diagnosis of dementia. In addition, the emphasis will be more upon the basic principles rather than a detailed examination of the validation data for each test that is mentioned. Those requiring to know the exact psychometric characteristics of any test are in any case best advised to look these up for themselves rather than to rely upon a second hand account. A further limitation in this section is that techniques like the Rorschach and other projective tests which rely largely upon a subjective analysis of the subject's response will be ignored. The basic justifications for this are that they have been infrequently used with demented patients, their demonstrated levels of validity are extremely poor, and the rationale for the use of projective tests in organic conditions of the brain is rather dubious because it is usually the non-orectic functions that are of most significance. A last point is that many of the diagnostic tests were originally designed to detect all forms of 'brain damage' and they will only be considered in relation to the very specific problem of dementia.

The diagnostic tests to be described below fall naturally into two groups. These first of these comprises tests based upon learning and/or memory. We have already seen that patients with dementia are appreciably impaired with regard to the learning and retention of new information and this has been exploited in diagnostic tests because patients with functional psychiatric disorders do not generally appear to be similarly impaired. The second group of tests are those which require the subject to reproduce geometric designs. The subject is usually asked to draw the design from memory but he may just have to copy the design that is in front of him. Again dements do badly on this type of task when compared with those who have functional psychiatric disorders. This may well be partly due to the involvement of memory but the disturbed perception of visuospatial relationships that occurs in dementia could well be the significant factor.

A common principle in learning/memory tasks has been to take a set of words whose meanings are unknown to the subject and to teach him the meanings of these words using a specified procedure. This principle was first proposed by Shapiro and Nelson (1955) but by far the best known test is the Modified World Learning Test of Walton and Black (1957). This is based on the vocabulary scale of one of the major intelligence tests and this scale is administered until the subject fails to give a scorable definition for 10 consecutive words. These 10 words then form the basis of the test proper and their selection in this way was designed to equalize the effects of different vocabulary levels. A possible weakness of the test is that the procedure for teaching the meanings of these 10 words is not very closely specified. Walton *et al.* (1959) later simplified the scoring of the test. These original reports, and a number of later ones (e.g., Bolton *et al.*, 1967), have agreed in showing that the test has a useful degree of validity. It correctly classifies a high proportion of those with functional psychiatric disorders as being without cerebral involvement and it also identifies the majority of those with organic disease of the brain. An important limitation of the Walton–Black test is that it results in an appreciable mis-classification of non-organic subjects when their intelligence level is in or near the range associated with mental retardation. (A similar limitation may be found for other learning tests of this type but the appropriate data are not always available).

A test similar to the Modified Word Learning Test and designed specifically for use with geriatric populations has been described by Kendrick *et al.* (1965). It is known as the Synonym Learning Test and is based on the Mill Hill Vocabulary Scale. It also has a more rigidly laid down procedure for teaching the meanings of words together with a different method of scoring. The Synonym Learning Test, unlike the other diagnostic tests to be described, does not stand on its own and it is necessary to administer a simple test of motor speed (the Digit Copying Test) with it.

Kendrick's approach to diagnostic discrimination has been more sophisticated than most in that he has used Bayesian statistics in the development of his small battery of tests (see Kendrick, 1965). The use of the Bayesian model enables the test user to take into account the fact that one diagnosis may be more likely than another in the normal clinical situation. For example, Kendrick has made the assumption that in the psychogeriatric populations for which the differential diagnosis between depression and dementia is appropriate, there is an antecedent probability that about 33% will be demented. Glaister (1971) has shown that this assumption is not unreasonable within a typical psychiatric hospital. Kendrick (1967) has cross validated his tests and shown that a diagnostic accuracy of up to 90% can be achieved using the Synonym Learning Test together with the Digit Copying Test.

Another test devised specifically for use with geriatric populations is the Inglis Paired Associate Learning Test. This test has two forms each of which consists of three pairs of unrelated words (e.g., Cabbage—Pen, Knife—Chimney, Sponge—Trumpet). The subject is required to learn the three associations by a similar procedure to that used in laboratory experiments on paired associate learning in normal subjects. Inglis (1959b) showed that this test gave a worthwhile level of discrimination between patients with and without clinically evident dementia. Cross-validation studies have been carried out (Caird *et al.*, 1962; Parsons, 1965) and these have confirmed Inglis' original claims.

The above comprise the main tests of learning and/or memory of major value in the differential diagnosis of dementia. There are, of course, a large number of other memory tests, some of which may also eventually prove to be of value in this context. Williams (1965) has reviewed in detail the many approaches to the measurement of memory in clinical practice. This endeavour need not be repeated here save to mention a small number of tests and techniques very briefly.

The Wechsler Memory Scale (Wechsler, 1945) has been used quite extensively and is still often found in the test repertoires of practising psychologists or used as a dependent variable in clinical research. Its protracted popularity stems both from its being an early stadardized test purporting to measure memory and because of its association with Wechsler's extremely successful intelligence scales. Unfortunately the Wechsler Memory Scale as a whole has been found to be inadequate. For example, Hall (1957) demonstrated that the reliability of the scale hardly exceeded that of the level of its correlation with the Wechsler–Bellevue Intelligence Scale. This implies that the scale's 'memory quotient' is not measuring anything that is much different from IQ. Specific subtests of the Wechsler Memory Scale, such as the one involving paired-associate learning, may have some potential for the diagnosis of dementia but the available standardization data is very poor and better alternatives are available.

A more sensibly designed set of memory tests than those included in the Wechsler Memory Scale has been presented by Williams (1968) who has also gone to the trouble of trying to provide three parallel forms. Later evaluative work carried out at another centre (White et al., 1969) has confirmed that one, at least, of William's subtests may have worthwhile diagnostic potential. This is the test of delayed recall. At the other extreme, the Rey–Davis test of non-verval learning, which is also a part of the battery, does not emerge very well from the investigation by White et al. The three alternative forms of the test battery also did not achieve intercorrelations that were high enough for them to be used interchangeably.

In general it can be claimed that some tests of learning and memory have proved capable of making a useful contribution to the differential diagnosis of dementia. Unfortunately those tests that have been shown to have worthwhile levels of validity also encounter practical difficulties. They are often tedious to administer and can prove distressing to the patient with a failing memory. The subject who cannot readily learn the definitions in a test like the Walton–Black Modified Word Learning Test may well recognize that he ought to be able to recall the meanings of the words that are repeatedly being defined for him. Such patients may refuse to continue with testing before the learning criterion is mastered or the diagnostic cut-off point is reached.

Future developments may lead to tests of learning and memory which are less stressful but equally effective. Pearce and Miller (1973) have advocated the use of tests based on the free recall technique whereby the subject is asked to recall words from a list and a fresh list is used on each trial. The use of free recall in an experimental situation (Miller, 1971) has shown that it is a much more acceptable method of testing memory than the approach involved in learning the meanings of new words. As yet uncompleted investigations by the present writer indicate that useful levels of validity may be obtained from a free recall test and that the test–re-test reliability is quite good. The high reliability is of significance since it may then be possible to develop an instrument which can adequately measure changes in memory over time.

A more radical development which has great potential is that of automated testing (Gedye and Miller, 1969, 1970; Miller, 1968). The essence of this is to use a teaching machine as a test administration device. This was found to be acceptable to even quite markedly deteriorated geriatric patients, many of whom were untestable by more conventional means. It is regrettable that this early promising work has not yet been systematically followed up to the point of providing a properly standardized test. A preliminary version of a learning test is available which has yielded some encouraging data as to its reliability and validity (Levy and Post, 1975), and which has been used with some success to evaluate cognitive changes in drug trials (Gedye et al., 1972).

The second major type of diagnostic test which can be used to discriminate dementia from functional psychiatric disorders is the design copying test. As has already been briefly indicated, the basic task which these tests exploit is very simple. The subject is merely required to copy (i.e., draw) a set of geometrical designs that he has been shown. This is usually from memory. The design is shown for a set time and then withdrawn before the subject attempts his copy but he may even be asked simply to copy a design that is before him all the time. A subtest of this type is included in the Wechsler Memory Scale but the best known of these tests are the Visual Motor Gestalt Test (Bender, 1946), the Revised Visual Retention Test (Benton, 1963) and Graham and Kendall's (1960) Memory-for-Designs Test.

It is unfortunate that much of the information relating to these tests has come from investigations which have examined their ability to discriminate between 'organic' and 'non-organic' groups of patients. The 'organic' groups contained patients with all types of brain disease including dementia. In a study of this type, Brilliant and Gynther (1963) used all three tests and obtained similar results for each. About two-thirds of the 'organics' were correctly identified and a very high proportion of a group with functional psychiatric disorders were correctly classified as 'non-organic'. However the discriminatory power was not so impressive when the data were corrected to allow for the much higher probability (about 0·70) that any given case would be 'non-organic'.

Although Crookes and McDonald (1972) do not present their data in a way that is very convenient for the crude assessment of discriminatory power, they appear to confirm that Benton's Revised Visual Retention Test is able to distinguish between dements and depressives at about the same level as was shown by Brilliant and Gynther (1963) for 'organics' and 'non-organics'. With regard to the Bender Visual Motor Gestalt Test there is very little information relating specifically to demented populations. Hain (1964) has attempted to develop a better scoring system for this test but this has not yet given better diagnostic validity than the original scoring system used in Brilliant and Gynther's (1963) investigation.

Scores on tests like these invariably also reflect variables other than the presence or absence of brain pathology. In the case of the Memory-for-Designs Test there are significant correlations between the raw score on the one hand and age or vocabulary level on the other. The correlation with vocabulary may well represent the influence of intelligence on the test score. The devisers of this test attempted to be rather more sophisticated than is usually the case by introducing special correction procedures to adjust the raw scores in order to try to eliminate the effects of age and vocabulary level. In view of this it is disappointing that later investigators (e.g., Alexander, 1970; Turland and Steinhard, 1969) have found that this correction procedure does not give a measure which has greater diagnostic power than the unadjusted raw score, and its use is therefore an unnecessary complication. In addition Alexander (1970) also found that the ability of the Memory-for-Designs Test to detect dementia in elderly populations was disappointing.

A further attempt to enhance the diagnostic validity of the design copying tests is illustrated by the use of the 'background interference procedure' with the Bender Gestalt Test. This utilizes the usual Bender designs but they are displayed against a background of intersecting curved lines. The use of this interfering background has been found to have little effect on the performance of normal subjects but it does have a very detrimental effect on that of demented patients (Canter and Straumanis, 1969).

On the whole the design copying tests do seem to have some discriminatory power. This is less impressive when base rates are taken into account (Brilliant and Gynther, 1963) and in any case these tests are not as useful as the tests of learning and memory. The one other thing in favour of the design copying tests is that they are quick and easy to administer and much less potentially stressful for the elderly patient than learning/memory tests.

NEUROPSYCHOLOGICAL EXAMINATION

Dementia can be associated with neuropsychological signs (aphasias, apraxias, etc.) rather like those found as a result of focal lesions in the brain. For this reason it can be useful to screen patients with a suspected dementia for these features. An immediate difficulty is that there is very little in the way of objective, standardized tests in this area and, for the most part, simple clinical techniques are all that can be carried out. An added complication is the lack of data to indicate how frequently the various signs may be encountered in either demented patients or those with functional psychiatric disorders. A single, partial exception is provided by the signs of extrapyramidal involvement for which Pearce and Miller (1973) have reported the incidence in a series of 50 patients with presenile dementia. Of the features looked for the most common was a positive glabella tap reflex which occurred in 46% of the sample.

Some suggestions with regard to the neuropsychological examination of the demented patient are given by Pearce and Miller (1973). Warrington (1970) also gives a more general account of the psychological examination of the neurological patient and many of the procedures that she describes are applicable in this context. In the writer's experience the most useful tests are those of language and praxis. These also have the virtue of being amongst the most easy to administer.

As we have seen in Chapter Five, disturbances of naming have been described in dementia and it is a very easy procedure to ask a patient to name a series of, say, 20 objects or pictures of objects. The available evidence also indicates that it is useful for some of the objects to have names that are not so commonly encountered in everyday speech providing that they still remain within the normal vocabulary of most members of the general population. Errors such as perseverations or failures to name are of obvious significance but undue delays in naming, even where the correct name is eventually supplied, may be a cause for suspicion with further testing being carried out as a check.

Tests of the understanding of language may also be useful. Potentially the best of these is the Token Test (De Renzi and Vignolo, 1962). This makes use of a set of 'tokens' of different shapes, sizes and colours which are set out in front of the subject. The subject is then asked to carry out instructions which are of increasing liguistic complexity (e.g., 'give me the blue circle' and 'put the small red rectangle on top of the large yellow circle'). This test is readily quantifiable but as yet there are no published normative data for dementia.

The other useful tests are those of praxis especially constructional apraxia. As has been argued elsewhere (Miller, 1972a; Warrington, 1970) constructional apraxia is almost certainly due to a disturbance in the appreciation of visuospatial relationships rather than a true apraxia, although this is more of an academic issue in the present situation. The easiest tests of constructional apraxia are those where the subject is required to draw things (e.g., a star or a three dimensional drawing of a cube). It is extremely difficult to develop norms for this type of test and so the tester has to rely on clinical experience in deciding what is abnormal. Another popular type of test of constructional apraxia utilizes Koh's blocks or their derivatives as in the Wechsler Block Design subtest.

Although neuropsychological tests often have to be interpreted on the unsatisfactory basis of clinical judgement, demented patients can sometimes respond in ways that are clearly outside the range for subjects without intracranial pathology. What these techniques cannot indicate with any certainty is whether the brain pathology is generalized, as in dementia, or of a more focal nature. Because these tests rely on clinical judgement, apparently positive results from their application are best regarded as merely suggestive unless the observed disturbances really are gross. In this case the patient may well be so demented that the diagnosis is not in doubt.

SOME TECHNICAL CONSIDERATIONS

An important feature of most differential diagnostic exercises is that the possible alternatives are usually not equiprobable. Within any particular unit the incidence of true cases of dementia amongst those referred for psychological examination, because of this possibility, may vary considerably. This incidence of a given diagnosis is known as the 'antecedent probability' or 'base rate'. The influence of the base rate on the clinical usefulness of a diagnostic test can be considerable.

The basic principles underlying the relationship between base rates, diagnostic validity and the decisions that can legitimately be made on the basis of a test, have been set out by Meehl and Rosen (1955). A useful but briefer description is also given by Gathercole (1968). The more mathematical aspects need not be repeated here but intuitively it can be appreciated that if the base rate is extreme, then a diagnostic test needs to have an unusually high validity to contribute any worthwhile information. For example, if 90% of those tested in order to try to discriminate between dementia and depression ultimately prove to be demented, then a 90% level of accuracy in diagnosis can be achieved simply by predicting that all tested patients are demented. A test would need to have an extremely high level of validity indeed to improve upon this. The maximum improvement in accuracy that could be attained is only 10% even given the unbelievable occurrence of a test with perfect validity.

The situation yielding maximum potential test usefulness is where the alternative diagnoses are equiprobable, i.e. the base rate for dementia is 50% where the discrimination is between dementia and a functional psychiatric disorder. Here the success of guessing is at a minimum and there is the maximum room for improvement. In this situation a test with only modest validity may give a worthwhile increment in diagnostic accuracy.

Very few test constructors and gathers of test data have taken base rates into account. The sole exception amongst the producers of the tests considered in this chapter is Kendrick (1965) with his Synonym Learning and Digit Copying Tests. Occasionally others have reworked existing norms taking base rates into account or they have restandardized established tests with this feature in mind. An example is Glaister (1971) who has dealth with the Walton–Black Modified Word Learning Test, the Benton Revised Visual Retention Test and the Graham–Kendall Memory-for-Designs Test. It is interesting that Kendrick's base rate for dementia in elderly patients referred in order to make a differentiation between in dementia and depression is 33%. This is very close to the base rate of 29% for 'brain damaged' individuals given by Glaister for patients in a very large psychiatric hospital who were investigated by the psychologist for possible evidence of brain damage. Of course the majority of 'brain damaged' patients encountered in this type of setting are dementias.

Another point of significance concerning the use of diagnostic tests involves the setting of cut-off points (i.e., the score below which a subject is considered to be, say, demented.) Most standardization data for tests is presented with a cut-off point which gives the maximum overall accuracy of diagnosis considering both alternatives together. In certain circumstances this may not be the most desirable choice. It could be argued that where the differentiation between dementia and depression is concerned it is particularly undesirable to fail to identify a case of depression and thus not deal appropriately with a treatable condition. Giving antidepressant medication by mistake to a demented patient might be considered a much less serious error. If this set of beliefs is held it might then be appropriate to shift the test cut-off point to a more stringent criterion for dementia. This would reduce the number of unidentified cases of depression at the expense of a larger proportion of misclassified dements and a slightly lower overall level of diagnostic accuracy.

The way in which many validation studies are conducted leads to limitations in the usefulness of the data. Quite often relatively unambiguous cases are used to form the groups on which a validation is carried out. Such groups may well not be representative of the general run of cases seen in the clinic; it is of course the patient with the ambiguous pattern of signs and symptoms who presents the diagnostic difficulty and for whom a special diagnostic test would have the greatest potential usefulness. A recent follow-up of cases originally diagnosed as having pre-senile dementia (Nott and Fleminger, 1975) shows that in many cases there is real cause to doubt this diagnosis at a later date. It is therefore desirable that diagnostic tests should be validated by administering them to exactly the same type of case that would be referred for testing should the test be of value. In addition, diagnoses should be established by carefully following the sample for a long enough period of time to establish these beyond doubt. So far, no diagnostic studies have adequately covered both these requirements.

Considerations of the type just described mean that it is not advisable to take published normative data for diagnostic tests and apply these without further consideration in another setting, or with a slightly different sample of patients. Unfortunately this is what clinical psychologists commonly do in practice. Rather, the local circumstances such as base rates should be investigated and the normative data adjusted accordingly. Better still is the development of local norms using data acquired with due regard to all the necessary principles of validation. This is too tedious for the majority of tests but there is no reason why psychology departments should not be able to manage this for their most commonly used diagnostic tests. The principle of developing local norms is not unique since it is common practice in many pathology laboratories.

As a final point there are limitations on the maximum validity that can be attained by any diagnostic test. Validity is impaired by a test's lack of perfect reliability but also because any psychological test in this field is inevitably not measuring the pathological process directly. The dementing illness impairs learning and it is learning that is measured by the test. The correlation between the pathological process and the degree of learning impairment will not be perfect and so, even if we could achieve the impossible and measure learning with complete accuracy, our test would still not correlate exactly with the disease process. Despite the fact that diagnostic tests may be of value in many circumstances these inevitable limitations mean that their use is not justified in others.

EXAMINING THE PATIENT WITH POSSIBLE DEMENTIA

The general approach to the psychometric assessment of the demented patient is not in principle different from that involved with any other type of adult patient. In some cases a little more attention needs to be given to some aspects of the procedure but these are obvious once time is taken to think about the situation. The demented patient may well be a little confused and not completely aware of what is happening. Mild communication difficulties are not uncommon and these can be compounded by the inevitable memory impairment. As a result, things need to be explained a little more slowly and carefully and, if necessary, repeated. The patient can also take a little longer than usual to settle down to testing and a failure to express anxieties about it should not be taken as indicating that he is happy with the situation. Patients with early dementia can be very much aware that they are not performing as well as they ought and therefore considerable tact is often needed as well as the judicious use of encouragement in order to maintain motivation.

A suggested procedure for the psychological examination of the demented patient is set out in Table 6. This assumes that the most important problem is distinguishing a possible dementia from a functional psychiatric disorder. The discrimination of a generalized neurological condition like dementia from focal lesions in the brain is rather more difficult. It relies mainly on neuropsychological testing to see if the deficits observed are confined to those associated with one part of the brain as would be expected in the case of a focal lesion. Dementia can produce signs associated with many different parts of the brain

TABLE 6

Summary of the psychological investigation of the patient suspected of having dementia. From Pearce and Miller (1973) by permission of Baillière Tindall

Stage	Information gained
1. Intelligence test (preferably Wechsler)	(a) Possible indication of intellectual deterioration (b) Base against which further changes can be measured
2. Dignostic tests (a) Learning tests (as appropriate for age)	Poor performance excludes functional disorder but is consistent with all other neurological conditions that produce severe amnesia
(b) Memory-for-designs test	May exclude functional disorder but results often equivocal
3. Neuropsychological examination for aphasia, aproxia, etc.	Positive findings indicate organic pathology
4. Retest on any cognitive test for which previous test results are available	Rarely possible but good indication of intellectual decline
5. Repeat all or part of stages 1 to 3 after several weeks	Evidence of progressive deterioration

and is not associated with visual field defects nor does it usually produce lateralized effects. It should also be stressed that psychological findings should not be considered in isolation but in the light of other types of information (neurological, radiological, psychiatric, etc.). The means available to other disciplines for the diagnosis of dementia are also far from foolproof and sound clinical practice must inevitably involve the weighing of one type of evidence against another.

9
The Management and Amelioration of Dementia

The demented patient is likely to survive for some time after the condition has become manifest (Shah *et al.*, 1969; Wang and Whanger, 1971). During this time there is the difficult problem of management and the possibility of amelioration of the symptoms needs to be explored. In the all too recent past the general approach to management has been one of therapeutic nihilism. The assumption, either explicit or implicit, has been that dementia is incurable and its effects irreversible. All that can be done is to look after the patient's basic needs as humanely as possible until nature takes its inevitable course. This attitude has recently started to change but it is only fair to note that there were a few (e.g., Cameron, 1941; Cosin *et al.*, 1958) who had thought beyond mere custodial management before the present trend to a more positive approach got under way.

Greater optimism about the management of dementia has come from two sources. Firstly there have been a number of medical and surgical treatments proposed which have been designed to halt, or even reverse, the pathological processes underlying some conditions associated with dementia. These have involved the insertion of by-pass 'shunts' for cerebrospinal fluid in so-called 'normal pressure hydrocephalus', hyperbaric oxygen treatment, and various pharmacological preparations. Secondly, there has been an encouraging interest in psychological and social methods of modifying the impact of dementia on the afflicted individual's general level of functioning. An indication of this growing interest in dementia and related problems in geriatric populations can be seen in the symposium on 'Psychological Involvement in Old Age' published in the Spring 1973 issue of *The Gerontologist*, a journal specifically concerned with new developments in the field of ageing.

The new medical approaches to the treatment of dementia are of peripheral importance to this volume with its emphasis on psychological aspects. Also they do not always relate directly to dementia associated with diffuse cortical atrophy. Despite this they cannot be entirely ignored because no one method of management can be completely evaluated without reference to any possible alternatives or supplementary techniques. In addition, it could be argued that the possibility of finding some way of halting the pathological progression of the disease adds emphasis to the need to find ways to help the afflicted individual cope with any residual incapacity. Because of this we will look briefly at the status of these medical developments before considering the social and psychological aspects of management in some detail.

MEDICAL TREATMENTS OF DEMENTIA

The newer medical approaches to the treatment or alleviation of the dementing illnesses will be outlined and a quick evaluation of their present position will be given. No attempt will be made to produce a comprehensive description of all the issues and many of these are beyond the range of competence of the present writer. The aim is merely to provide background information about the various medical developments which could affect the overall management of dementia.

Normal Pressure Hydrocephalus

Hydrocephalus is a condition which in most peoples minds is more commonly associated with children but it can occur in adults. It happens most commonly when there is a blockage in the circulation of cerebrospinal fluid (CSF) or a failure to absorb CSF. The consequence of this is that the pressure of CSF within the ventricles of the brain increases and this causes the ventricles to be forced out and enlarged. In babies before the age at which the bones in the skull have become fused the pressure will also cause the head to expand but this is not possible in adults where the skull has fused and has become a rigid container for the brain. Hydrocephalus can be treated surgically by means of a shunt which draws off CSF from within the ventricles and returns it to the blood stream outside the skull.

Hakim and Adams (1965) and Adams *et al.* (1965) reported the successful surgical treatment of alleged hydrocephalus in adult patients with signs of dementia who also had normal CSF pressures. As a result the concept of 'normal pressure hydrocephalus' was born. It is assumed that some patients owe their dementia to a situation in which the normal CSF pressure has become too much and therefore produces the effect of a hydrocephalus within the brain. There seems to be no satisfactory explanation as to why the normal CSF pressure should become excessive and cause a hydrocephalus. One suggestion is that the normal changes in the brain with ageing, e.g. the loss of cells, might cause brain tissue to be less able to withstand the usual CSF pressure levels. Regardless of the mechanism involved it is alleged that cases of normal pressure hydrocephalus show the characteristic hydrocephalic pattern of ventricular enlargement with little or no cortical atrophy and that the expected CSF dynamics can be demonstrated when the appropriate radiological investigations are undertaken.

The concept of normal pressure hydrocephalus was taken up with enthusiasm in many centres because it presented the possibility of identifying one subgroup of demented patients that could be treated surgically with some success. Recent reviews of the topic (Benson, 1974; Wood *et al.*, 1974) indicate that the basic issues are still not clear. There is appreciable disagreement about the appropriate diagnostic criteria and the ways in which normal pressure hydrocephalus can be distinguished from the ordinary type of cerebral atrophy. Clinically it is claimed that normal pressure hydrocephalus is more likely to be associated with a relatively sudden onset of the dementia and the occurrence of ataxia and incontinence. These are hardly very reliable indices. The radiological criteria are clear in principle but do not reliably predict response to surgery.

The clinical trials of the insertion of shunts in supposed cases of normal pressure hydrocephalus are not impressive with regard to their methodological sophistication, and give very mixed outcomes which range from a very high proportion of patients with improved functioning to results that are definitely disappointing. Most centres seem to have had a few dramatic successes and a good number of cases that were either total failures or showed very little change. It remains a possibility that better definition of the syndrome may lead to an effective method of treating a small proportion of cases that fit into the general category of dementia with cerebral atrophy. Even so it still remains to be seen to what extent a successful operation can lead towards a complete recovery of lost functional capacity and whether a single shunt operation can give satisfactory long-term control.

Hyperbaric Oxygen

Jacobs *et al*. (1969) exposed aged persons with intellectual deficits to 100% oxygen at a pressure of 2·5 atmospheres for a total of 3 hours per day over 15 days. They claimed an almost uniformally beneficial response as indicated by improved psychological test performance in their 27 patients. Unfortunately the effects were only transient but, if the results can be confirmed, it raises the hope that more extensive treatment could produce longer lasting changes. A further examination of this form of treatment has been made by Goldfarb *et al*. (1972). Goldfarb and his colleagues treated a smaller series of patients consisting both of cases of senile dementia and those with cerebral vascular disease, using a similar therapeutic regime to that of Jacobs *et al*. Subjects were evaluated before, during, and after treatment by a multidisciplinary team which included a neurologist, a psychiatrist and a psychologist. The separate evaluations all agreed in showing no improvements in social or intellectual functioning. The treatment was also disliked by the patients and only two thirds managed to complete the full course. Further investigations are needed but the most sensible attitude for the present is one of healthy scepticism. The history of therapeutic endeavour shows that initial enthusiastic reports on the basis of uncontrolled trials are commonly followed by a failure to repeat the success when subjected to more detailed scrutiny.

Pharmacological methods

It has been suggested that ribonucleic acid (RNA) might be a substrate of memory (e.g., Hydén, 1955). Work on this hypothesis has produced negative results in some instances but there is also a substantial amount of evidence which is consistent with it (Hydén, 1970). An obvious step from this theory is to see if the administration of RNA would be of benefit in those clinical conditions for which a defect in memory could be considered an important feature.

The first attempts to test out RNA on the disorders of ageing were carried out in Montreal by Cameron and his associates (Cameron, 1958; Cameron and Solyom, 1961; Cameron et al., 1963). Various groups of elderly subjects were treated by the administration of RNA and evaluated in a number of ways which included the administration of tests like the Wechsler Memory Scale. It was claimed that a substantial proportion of cases showed a good response. Those with arteriosclerotic dementia did best and RNA was least effective in patients with senile dementia. Subjects with pre-senile dementia responded at a level mid way between the other two groups. It is regrettable that these early studies did not employ control groups. It is well established that subjects often perform much better on their second exposure to psychometric tests and such practice effects could well have accounted for the improved scores that Cameron and his colleagues obtained.

As is all too often the case that better controlled trials fail to show any therapeutic effect. Britton et al. (1972) used a cross-over design to test RNA against placebo in hospitalized patients with severe memory defects (the sample was not defined any better than this but the majority of patients with marked memory impairments in a typical psychiatric hospital would be demented). RNA had no detectable effect on the learning or retention of paired associates. Similarly Munch-Petersen et al. (1974) found no beneficial effect of RNA over placebo in a conventional double blind trial. These and other findings leave very little confidence in the value of RNA.

The most extensively advocated pharmacological treatment has been the use of cerebrovascular dilators. These are drugs intended to produce dilatation of the cerebral blood vessels and would be expected to be of benefit to demented patients for whom an inadequate blood supply to the brain could be considered a significant aetiological factor. This is especially the case for arteriosclerotic dementia but there are a few who would extend the potential value of these drugs to other types of dementia.

Of the steadily increasing varieties of these drugs we shall only deal with one example but this is the one that appears to have been subjected to the most careful evaluation. Cyclandelate (Cyclospasmol) has been shown to cause dilatation of cerebral blood vessels and to increase cortical perfusion rates (Eichorn, 1965; O'Brien and Veall, 1966). Unlike most of the alternative preparations cyclandelate has been subjected to a number of reasonably well designed trials in order to demonstrate its efficacy in producing changes in mental functioning.

Ball and Taylor (1967) report a double-blind trial in which cyclandelate was tested against a placebo. The subjects were elderly patients in long-term care in a geriatric unit. The sample was not very well described but it seems that the subjects were demented to some degree although not so much as to make simple mental testing impossible. If the sample was relatively unselected apart from these criteria it would be expected that many of the subjects would be straightforward cases of senile dementia. The drug was found to enhance performance on mental tests, most of which were clinical in nature, but which did include a more formal test of memory. The drug also increased cerebral blood flow. On the other hand there was no correlation between changes in blood flow and changes on the mental tests. As the authors point out this implies that the benefit arises not simply just as a result of increased blood flow and they suggest that it is possibly a more effective distribution of the flow within the brain that is the crucial factor.

Trials using patients with definite arteriosclerotic dementia have also produced positive results. Fine *et al.* (1970) carried out a double-blind cross-over trial and showed that cyclandelate produced significant improvement in some of the mental tests they employed. In particular these were measures of orientation and digit span. In a similar experiment with longer treatment periods and extending over a year instead of the 4 months of Fine *et al.*, Young *et al.* (1974) observed that administration of a placebo was associated with a decline in functioning whilst the active preparation maintained the initial levels on a number of measures including some derived from the Wechler Adult Intelligence Scale.

There is therefore evidence from reasonably well conducted trials that at least one drug claimed to be a cerebral vasodilator (cyclandelate) can halt, and even possibly partially reverse, the decline in mental functions caused by arteriosclerotic dementia. It may well be that other drugs of this type will prove to have similar effects. There are already a number of claims for other preparations but the evidence on which these are based comes from trials designed. Even where such things as double-blind procedures have been used the value of the investigation has been reduced by confused data analysis (Bouvier *et al.*, 1974). So far there is only good support for the beneficial effects of drugs in the case of arteriosclerotic dementia. In view of Ball and Taylor's (1967) report, which may have been based at least partially on subjects with senile dementia, further well designed and executed trials might well be warranted for this latter condition.

General Comment on Medical Developments

It would be presumptuous of this author to speculate on any further trends in the medical management of dementia. This brief survey has demonstrated that it is not beyond the bounds of possibility that the progress of some dementing illnesses might be halted or even possibly reversed. These medical developments help to modify the usual pessimistic attitude towards the management of dementia and, as already indicated, they give an added impetus to the need to find ways of helping the afflicted individual to cope with his handicaps. Behavioural approaches to management, which form the main topic of this chapter, cannot be fully evaluated unless they are also studied in combination with the appropriate medical treatments where these are applicable.

PSYCHOLOGICAL AND PSYCHOSOCIAL METHODS OF MANAGEMENT

Although there are some earlier exceptions, the general idea that the problems of dementia might be modifiable by environmental manipulations has only achieved wide currency within the last decade. Amongst clinical psychologists Inglis (1962) was one of the first to advocate that the psychologist should step beyond the questions of evaluation and measurement and try to intervene in an active way in order to achieve therapeutic goals. At this stage Inglis was largely forced to state what he thought ought to be done rather than describe what had been demonstrated to be of value. He was able to cite a small amount of previous work (Cameron, 1941; Cosin *et al.*, 1958; Sommer and Ross, 1958) showing that even confused senile patients were sensitive to environmental features. In another article whose tone was necessarily prescriptive rather than descriptive, Lindsley (1964) presented the notion of the 'prosthetic environment'. By this he meant an environment which is specifically designed to fit in with the behavioural limitations of the elderly. Both Inglis and Lindsley were writing about the problems of old age in general but their ideas are as applicable to dementia as to any other form of incapacity in old age.

In dealing with the psychological aspects of management we shall first review reports of the consequences of making various social and psychological manipulations on the behaviour of demented patients. This will have the effect of marshalling the evidence for the validity of a psychological approach to management and possibly give some indication of what techniques are likely to be most effective in attaining certain goals. This will then lead to a discussion of the particular techniques that are available or have been used so far. Finally there will be some speculation on the ways in which this very recent field of endeavour might develop together with an appraisal of some of its likely problems and limitations.

Effects of Psychological and Social Intervention

From a historical point of view the first worker in this area (or at least the first to gain any recognition) was Cameron (1941). He studied the wandering confusion that some senile patients show at night and discovered that the same disorganized behaviour could be produced in daytime by placing the patient in a darkened room. This led to the conclusion that confusion was a function of the level of background stimulation. Cameron speculated that his senile patients could not maintain a spatial image in the absence of repeated visual stimulation. Unfortunately Cameron does not report having taken the issue any further but this paper is a landmark in demonstrating that an undesirable symptom can be brought under the control of environmental factors.

It was almost two decades before anything further of note was published. Sommer and Ross (1958) measured the amount of social interaction in a geriatric ward of which just over two thirds of the residents were demented.

Arranging the chairs into small groups around tables enhanced the amount of social interaction as compared with the previous level when the chairs were placed in l'ong lines. At about the same time, Cosin *et al.* (1958) were looking at the efficacy of social and occupational therapy when used with demented patients. Patients receiving such therapies responded by producing more appropriate behaviour. The most powerful effect was in increasing the amount of intercommunication within the patient group.

There was then very little interest for about another decade but since the late 1960s there has been a steady stream of reports of attempts to make direct interventions in the problems of confused and demented elderly patients. The extent of this surge of interest can be seen in the symposium on psychological intervention published in *The Gerontologist* in 1973. A considerable number of different therapeutic techniques have been suggested and these have been reviewed by Barns *et al.* (1973). As might be expected in an early phase of development, most authors are reporting their impressions of applying new techniques and so far there have been very few controlled trials.

Simple alterations in the pattern of ward activities have been claimed to produce beneficial effects. Bowers *et al.* (1967) organized special discussion groups and reported improvements in the group and general social behaviour of the demented old people who took part. Mueller and Atlas (1972) also had small discussion groups. Following baseline measurements, participants were given reinforcers (initially primary reinforcers like sweets but later tokens) which were contingent upon speaking. Increased verbal activity was recorded in the group setting and ward staff alleged that they could detect a carry over effect on the amount of verbal interaction in the general ward setting. Quilitch (1974) preferred to introduce a communal activity (playing Bingo). As compared with the initial baseline period, the time during which Bingo sessions were held was associated with increased 'purposeful activity'. Puposeful activity was defined in terms of talking to other patients and staff, using recreational materials provided on the ward, etc. However, once the Bingo sessions were discontinued this type of puposeful activity returned to its initial, very low level.

Folsom (1967) has advocated the use of 'reality orientation programmes' (an outline of this technique will be given later) and described some initial encouraging responses in individual patients. Barnes (1974) tried to apply the technique to 12 severely demented patients and found no change in the subjects' responses to a questionnaire designed to measure orientation. This paper is of interest in that it is the only essentially negative report of the effects of psychological intervention although it is possible that others have had a similar lack of success but failed to publish their findings. Barnes does offer the consolation that the nursing staff gained the impression that the patients had improved, but probably of greater significance is the fact that this was a group of very advanced cases.

An approach based on a theoretical notion has come from Bower (1967). He assumed that some of the symptoms of senile dementia were the result of sensory deprivation. Following on from this idea, he exposed a group of elderly dements to 'structured stimulation' for several hours a day over a period of 6 months. The 'structured stimulation' is inadequately described but seems to have consisted of an active attempt to get the subjects to participate in a variety of everyday tasks and recreational activities. As compared with a control group, the stimulated patients showed some changes in psychiatric state and in ratings made by occupational therapists.

If the work surveyed so far is to be believed, the introduction of different activities is likely to lead to improvements in behaviour especially in the areas of social and verbal interaction. It could be argued that what the various interventions have in common is that they increase directly or indirectly the level of social stimulation. The most plausible tentative conclusion that can be drawn is that increasing the level of social stimulation in institutionalized demented patients will enhance the quantity and quality of their social interactions.

There is a serious difficulty with these observations and that is that they are largely based on investigations that are either uncontrolled or poorly controlled. A few have taken baseline measures to compare with their treatment effects (e.g., Mueller and Atlas, 1972; Quilitch, 1974), and Bower (1967) actually had a control group. Despite this not even the best of these experiments could be considered as meeting the methodological criteria usually regarded as necessary for an acceptable clinical trial. For this reason the two methodologically purer investigations described below are of special interest.

In what is the most detailed single investigation carried out in this area so far, a research group in Philadelphia compared two matched groups of mentally-impaired, aged subjects (Brody et al., 1971, 1974; Kleban and Brody, 1972; Kleban et al., 1971). Both groups lived in similar accommodation in a geriatric centre and were extensively evaluated by a multidisciplinary team at the commencement and at successive stages of the project. In both groups an attempt was made to identify 'excess disabilities' (the occurrence of functional impairments judged to be in excess of those necessarily occurring as a result of the individuals organic condition). The experimental group then received individual treatment programmes aimed at reducing these excess disabilities.

The one major weakness of the published accounts is that the techniques used in these programmes and the criteria used to identify excess disabilities are not described in sufficient detail to give anything more than the vaguest idea of what was involved.

A number of fairly clear cut findings emerged. At the end of a year's treatment period, evaluation of the excess disabilities showed a very definite advantage in favour of the experimental group. After a further 9 months follow-up, this difference had been eroded away. The groups did not differ at any point on a wide range of other variables and both groups showed a decline in their general health over the year of the treatment period. This latter finding indicates that improvements in general health are not necessary prerequisites for improvement in excess disabilities and these can even be obtained in the presence of adverse changes in general health. A number of possible predictors of improvement were examined, especially various personality characteristics, but the only one that emerged with any appreciable correlation was aggressiveness.

The other well controlled trial is that of Brook *et al.* (1975) who attempted to assess the value of special reality orientation procedures. The experimental group was introduced to a special room over a 16-week period in which therapists actively engaged them in various tasks using materials in the room (e.g., describing objects, and writing a diary). The control group had a similar amount of exposure to the experimental room and its materials but the therapists remained passive and any activity had to be patient initiated. Ratings of intellectual and social functioning improved over the first 2 to 4 weeks in both groups but further gains after this time were confined to the experimental group. After their early improvement the control group began to fall back. This experiment implies that sustained benefits cannot be achieved merely by exposing patients to a different and possibly more visually stimulating environment. Active participation by the subjects and encouragement by the therapists is required if the initial improvements are to be built upon and not dissipated. The authors also report a general impression that the less severely demented patients gave the best responses. If this is so it would at least partially explain why Barnes (1974) found no effects of reality orientation in his advanced cases.

The large number of basically uncontrolled, or very poorly controlled, observations have thus been vindicated by two methodologically purer trials. This gives greater confidence as to the potential value of future work in this area. Following on from this a number of more detailed questions need to be asked. In general we need to know what specific procedures are likely to be effective, together with the results that they can be expected to achieve and the characteristics of patients that are most likely to show a good response. So far there are no more than a few hints about possible answers for these specific questions.

It is not really possible to say very much at this stage about the nature of effective techniques. A number of different procedures have been claimed to be of benefit but the literature is generally weak when it comes to describing the exact nature of what was done with the subjects. All attempted programmes have in common the provision of enhanced stimulation, but the work of Brook *et al.* (1975) shows that this is not always enough in itself for a lasting response. It is necessary for staff to ensure that the patients become actively involved in the situation. Further trials after the model of Brook *et al.* which systematically vary the nature of the therapeutic situation are needed to pinpoint the crucial features.

The beneficial effects that might be expected to follow from social and psychological interventions are also difficult to specify. It has already been noted that increased verbal behaviour and improved social interactions are the things that have been most commonly reported. The work of the Philadelphia group (Brody *et al.*, 1971) suggests that a variety of specific target symptoms can be attacked with some success but further details were not reported. Knowing what can be achieved is obviously a most important consideration in deciding which patients to work with in any therapeutic programme.

A related issue is knowing what aspects of the everyday behaviour of demented patients are most likely to become disrupted and which will therefore become a potential target for therapeutic intervention. Again, there is remarkably little information on this point. In one survey, Ferm (1974) noted that early on in the illness demented patients tended to lose the ability to wash and dress themselves reliably and also ceased to participate in hobbies and related recreational activities. In contrast, things like orientation in space, bowel control and the ability to recognize persons remained reasonably intact until well on in the illness.

An important aspect of the effectiveness of therapeutic programmes is the permanence of any changes. In a condition like dementia which is the result of a steady unchecked process within the brain, all gains are likely to be lost ultimately and so the real issue becomes whether they can be maintained for long enough to be worthwhile. In all those investigations in which an attempt has been made to see what happens after any special intervention has been discontinued, the finding has been that the beneficial effects are quickly dissipated (Brody *et al.*, 1974; Cosin *et al.*, 1958; Quilitch, 1974). This is not encouraging but it would be too pessimistic to conclude that gains are always too short lasting to be worth the effort expended in achieving them. Rather it indicates that, for the main part, social and psychological intervention must not be seen as a form of therapy in the usual sense, i.e. as an intervention which is made to correct some inadequacy and then withdrawn as soon as the objective is achieved. What is probably more appropriate is to think in terms of devising a permanent environment for the demented patient which will both produce and maintain more desirable behaviour for the rest of the patient's life. It is necessary to think of Lindsley's (1964) prosthetic environment instead of planning time-limited therapeutic interventions.

There is some tentative information regarding the types of demented patient most likely to benefit from a reorganized environment. Although the numbers involved were not large, Brook *et al.* (1975) observed a general trend towards a better response from the less severely demented subjects. This finding is in need of replication but is not at variance with common sense expectations. It is also in line with Barnes' (1974) failure to obtain any benefits from applying reality orientation principles to advanced cases. Kleban *et al.* (1971) examined a number of personality variables and concluded that the only predictor of response to their manipulations was the rated level of aggressiveness. In most applied settings personality factors have not emerged as very powerful predictors of anything and so cross-validation would be essential before this finding could be considered of value. This is particularly so as the design of the Kleban *et al.* investigation was such that one of the many variables might have been expected to throw up a spuriously high correlation by chance.

Specific Management Techniques

Although there is very little hard evidence as to which management procedures are most likely to be of value in dementia, a number of different approaches have been articulated and there are others that might be expected to be of value on *a priori* grounds. Barns *et al.* (1973) briefly describe a large number of techniques thought to be suitable for aged populations in general. Not all of these seem to be equally applicable to dementia and others are really variations on a more basic theme. Here discussion will be confined to the major methods of potential value for demented patients.

Reality Orientation

This may well be the first psychological technique specifically designed for use with the mentally-deteriorating aged. We are informed by Barns *et al.* (1973) that reality orientation procedures were initiated by Folsom at an American Veterans Administration Hospital in Kansas as early as 1958 but descriptions did not appear in the literature until some considerable time later (Folsom, 1967, 1968; Taulbee and Fosom, 1966). A useful summary and outline of the literature on this technique is also given by Barns *et al.* (1973). The essence of reality orientation is to ensure that the patient re-learns if necessary and then continually rehearses essential information relating to his orientation for time, place and person. Knowing the names and uses of commonly encountered objects and environmental features is also usually included. Reality orientation is promulgated in two ways. There are formal daily classes which may take place in a special room. In these the therapist rehearses patients in the appropriate types of information. The informal aspects go on all the time and rely on members of staff who come into contact with the patients stressing the same sort of basic information. For example, the night nurse approaching a restless patient in the early hours of the morning might normally say 'Is anything the matter?'. If the nurse is using reality orientation procedures she would stress the 'who' and 'when' of the situation by saying something like 'It is 2 o'clock in the morning. Is anything the matter Mrs Smith?'

As we have already seen, there is one controlled trial that attests to the efficacy of reality orientation procedures (Brook *et al.*, 1975) even though it does not reveal all the key features of the procedures. In its basic principles, reality orientation is easy to understand and use and can be readily communicated to the wide range of staff likely to come into direct contact with the patient. They can then carry out the informal aspects of the procedure by merely altering their verbal interactions with the patients in an appropriate manner. One obvious difficulty is that ward staff often change round rapidly and for this reason it may be difficult to achieve consistency in the informal application of the procedures. It seems likely that some inconsistency in the application of the principles would not be as serious a problem as is the case in using behaviour modification programmes. Finally there is an important question that advocates of reality orientation do not seem to have addressed themselves to. We have no sound evidence with regard to what information is essential for the elderly patient if he is to function at a reasonable level. The tacit assumption has been that this is obvious and to some extent this assumption may be justified. On the other hand it is also probable that empirical investigations of this point might throw up some unexpected findings.

Behaviour Modification

This is the application of operant conditioning principles and procedures to the modification of patient behaviour. One of the first advocates of its use with geriatric populations was Lindsley (1964), and behaviour modification has had considerable success in other clinical fields such as the management of chronic schizophrenics and the mentally retarted. This success in other fields has not yet led to psychologists skilled in behaviour modification being particularly active with the aged although there are a few reports which suggest that behaviour modification may become more extensively used with geriatric populations (e.g., Hoyer, 1973; Hoyer *et al.*, 1974). Specific applications to demented subjects are more difficult to document. Mueller and Atlas (1972) in the study described earlier, did use reinforcement principles to increase verbal interaction in a discussion group, and Libb and Clements (1969) have claimed that the use of tokens as reinforcers helped to increase the amount of effort put into physical excercises by a small group of demented patients.

The lack of any significant evidence restricts the usefulness of any consideration of behaviour modification techniques but the information that we do have shows that behaviour modification is of enough potential benefit to warrant being carefully examined. The apparent success of behaviour modification in another allegedly difficult area of therapeutic endeavour, mental retardation (e.g., Kiernan, 1974), supports this view. The basic principles of behaviour modification are too well known to need describing yet again and a number of excellent accounts are readily available (e.g., Kazdin, 1975). These principles are relatively simple and straightforward (at least at an elementary level) and so can be readily communicated to primary care staff such as nurses for application on the ward or other living unit. A major problem in running behaviour-modification programmes in any context lies in ensuring that all staff who come into contact with the patient follow the requirements of the programme in a consistent manner. The often rapid changeover of staff in living units makes this difficult but the difficulty has been overcome in other situations and can no doubt be similarly overcome on wards containing demented patients.

It can be anticipated that another appreciable difficulty in the use of behaviour-modification programmes with demented subjects will be in maintaining any functional improvements that are attained. This has already emerged as a common problem in the use of behaviour modification in other clinical settings (e.g., Kazdin, 1973, 1975). It is even more likely here in view of the already noted propensity for the effects of other types of intervention to be rapidly dissipated once the special manipulations have been withdrawn. Again the answer is likely to lie in building behaviour modification principles into the permanent features of the environment. In this way the necessary reinforcement contingencies for the maintenance of appropriate behaviour will always be present, unlike the situation where time-limited interventions are devised to deal with specific difficulties as they appear. The staff in the living units should always ensure that such things as self-care behaviour and social interaction are always reinforced and not just try to introduce reinforcement principles once the behaviour has broken down. It is unfortunately very easy to reinforce dependent behaviour in handicapped individuals. For example, the nurse who helps the patient to dress may actually reinforce a future lack of dressing because the patient welcomes the undivided attention from the nurse that being dressed entails. In dementia, more than almost any other handicapping condition, it is probably true that prevention by the maintenance of appropriate behaviour is likely to be far easier than curing the situation once that behaviour has broken down.

So far this discussion of behaviour modification has omitted an extremely important advantage which distinguishes behaviour modification from most alternative forms of psychological intervention. This is its inherent flexibility. A look at the use of behaviour modification with the severely retarded (e.g., Kiernan, 1974) shows that it can be used on a wide range of self-care, educational, occupational and social skills with even the most severely handicapped populations. This alone must go a long way to ensuring that behaviour modification will be an essential part of the professional repertoire of anyone wishing to intervene effectively in the management of demented patients by psychological means.

Ergonomics

Although he did not actually use the term, Lindsley (1964) wrote about issues with a strong ergonomic flavour in his discussion of possible means of enhancing the functional capacities of the elderly. For example, with advanced ageing the hands become less steady and the individual becomes less capable of excercising fine motor control. This tendency is almost certainly enhanced in dementia since there is evidence of poor performance on motor tasks (Miller, 1974a). Lindsley pointed out that this has implications for the design of electrical equipment and other tools. Button switches should require firmer pressure in order to avoid being activated by accidental contact and their size should be increased to make them more easily touched by a finger whose movements are not so accurately controlled.

To some degree the basic aims of an ergonomic approach have been used for some time. Occupational therapists have devised special implements to help the infirm carry out everyday functions like dressing and feeding. Some designers of units which may house confused or elderly patients have added special cues to the environment. An example is in placing colour coded lines along the floors of corridors and some rooms. A resident who has great difficulty in remembering which way to go within the building then merely has to remember what colour line to follow to arrive at a desired goal such as the lavatory or dining room.

It is therefore apparent that thinking along ergonomic lines is not new and certainly not confined to those with special qualifications in psychology or ergonomics. Nevertheless the process of adapting environmental features to the behavioural limitations and peculiarities of confused and demented patients has probably not be taken as far as it could be by the application of the more sophisticated and scientific approach of ergonomics.

Normalization

The way of thinking embedded in normalization as a formal set of principles first arose in Sweden and other Scandinavian countries with respect to the management of the mentally retarded. The ideas then crossed the Atlantic and took root in the retardation services in Nebraska and elsewhere (see Wolfensberger, 1972). Normalization principles have now been extended to other fields concerned with the management of individuals whose behaviour is somehow deviant from societal norms. Wolfensberger (1970) has outlined the possible place of normalization principles in general psychiatry. So far there has been no specific statement with regard to psychogeriatrics although the principles are equally applicable in this field.

In outline, normalization is two things. Firstly it gives a goal. This goal is that of achieving a lifestyle and pattern of behaviour that is as near the society norm for the afflicted individual's normal peers as is possible. Most professionals working with handicapped groups of any kind would probably subscribe to this goal, but what distinguishes the advocates of normalization is the way in which they have thought through the implications of adopting this goal and the determination with which they have pursued it. The other aspect of normalization is that it is a principle of management. In simple outline it involves keeping those needing special care within an environment that is as close as can be achieved to the normal environment. It must be presumed that the normal environment acts so as to maintain normal patterns of behaviour and it can be confidently expected that abnormal environments are likely to produce abnormal behaviour. Normalization therefore places a very heavy stress on trying to ensure that handicapped individuals live in the community wherever possible. Where community living cannot be maintained, institutional living units must be designed by using society's normal living units as a model. On the other hand, the sensible use of normalization principles does not deny that residential environments for handicapped groups may need some special features that are atypical for the population at large. These must merely be kept to a minimum and only introduced to cope with some special need that a particular handicapped group has.

As far as the confused and demented patient is concerned, normalization implies that he must be managed in such a way that his life style deviates as little as possible from that of normal elderly persons. Long-term admission to an institution must be delayed for as long as is reasonably possible. Although its effects have not been systematically studied, it may be the case that occasional short-term admissions to enable the rest of the family to do such things as go on holiday, could make more families willing to look after a confused elderly relative at home. When the patient comes into residential care this should ideally have certain features. Normal old people do not normally live in large, sex segregated living units far from the usual residential areas and in which special management personnel, e.g. nurses, make everyday decisions for them (what to eat, when to eat, when to have a bath, etc.). In contrast the ideal living units should be small, have the sexes integrated and be situated within the usual residential areas of the community. They should ensure the maximum participation of residents in running their daily lives. A further implication of this last point is that staff levels should be kept to a minimum and this is a view which contrasts with the perennial complaint that there are never anything like enough primary care staff to go round. More staff are presumably needed so as better to order residents lives for them and it is not implausible that an excess of staff is likely to destroy rather than maintain any residual capacity for independent functioning that the residents might still retain. It must also be allowed that, in the case of a condition like dementia which is marked by a slow deterioration, there will have to be a steady transfer of control of his life from the patient to those taking care of him. The normalization principle stresses that this transfer should be as slow as possible and not accelerated by a situation which actually encourages his ever increasing dependence.

Final Comments on Management

There is no doubt that the increasing trend in clinical work with the demented patient is towards management and away from the more traditional concerns of assessment and classification. The evidence surveyed gives an encouraging indication that social and psychological methods for the maintenance of higher levels of functioning, and hopefully a better quality of life, are being developed. There are also some hopeful preliminary developments on the medical front which make it not unreasonable to expect that at least some dementing illnesses may eventually have their progress arrested by drugs and other means.

An important issue that must not be avoided in any discussion of the management of the dementing patient is that of the ethics of intervention. Why interfere in a situation where the individual's capacity is fading and he is nearing the termination of his life? Would he not be better off being cared for in a comfortable and humane environment which makes minimal demands and in which he is not being put under pressure by over enthusiastic management procedures? As Looft (1973) argues in his discussion of similar issues, there is no question of not intervening because everything that is done for the demented patient constitutes some form of intervention. What is needed is to set out clearly the goals of any action and the assumptions upon which they are based. Only then does it become sensible to discuss the ethics of various methods of management and in particular whether these should be active or essentially passive and undemanding.

In this writer's opinion the normalization principle is useful here. The handicapped older person, whether this handicap is a dementing illness or something else, would probably live like a normal member of society of his age level if he did not have the handicap. We have also seen from discussion of the disengagement theory in normal ageing (see Chapter 2) that old age is probably not ideally viewed as a time of complete withdrawal and it is quite normal to maintain some outside involvement in old age. In the absence of compelling evidence to the contrary, it seems quite reasonable to suppose that the dementing elderly person will be happiest in fulfilling, as far as he is able, the same sort of role and life style as his less handicapped peer.

Another important factor is that many of the manipulations that appear to have some effect do not directly put pressure on the patient in any way. Making the general environment more stimulating and better adapted to patients' needs and getting staff to use reality orientation principles in their interactions with them, make no extra demands from the patients' point of view. Operant conditioning procedures may interfere much more directly but experience suggests that if they are used with common sense and understanding they need not cause any distress in most cases. Even so a strong case could be made out to the effect that some temporary disturbance is justified if it results in the patient being better placed to control his own life in the future.

A final concern is that the discussions of management have been almost entirely conducted with regard to the institutionalized patient living in a hospital ward or other special facility. Many early cases continue to live in the community and some are looked after to quite an advanced stage by relatives (Kay et al., 1964a). In such cases the problems of management may be even more pressing to those providing the primary care than they are for hospital personnel who can at least retreat from the situation when not on duty. In addition the family home is not designed to take into account the needs of the confused older person. Keeping the dementing individual at home fits in well with the normalization principle but it is necessary that the strain placed on relatives and others should not be too great. The management of the demented patient in the community therefore needs some urgent attention. Any ways of making it easier to keep those afflicted with dementia, especially the milder cases, at home or otherwise in the community is likely to have the double benefit of slowing down the loss of functional capacity and also reducing the very heavy demand for psychogeriatric beds.

Part Four
Conclusions

10
Abnormal Ageing—Retrospect and Prospect

This book has proceeded in stages. Firstly the nature of dementia and the problems that it presents were defined. Next the psychological changes associated with normal ageing were outlined because these must necessarily be part of the total picture produced by dementia. The main chapters of the book have described the principal psychological changes recorded in dementia and an attempt has also been made to relate the psychological features to other manifestations of dementia (radiological, pathological, etc.). Some consideration was then given to the theoretical and practical issues surrounding dementia.

The discussion has ranged over a large variety of different topics. No general summary will be attempted since this would either be long and repetitive if it were to do justice to what has gone before, or oversimplified to the point of travesty if it were to be kept to a reasonable length. Instead it is intended to use this concluding chapter to do two things. Firstly it will pick up and elaborate upon some of the more general issues that have emerged from the previous chapters but which could not be readily dealt with at the time. Secondly, it is intended to speculate upon the way that psychological work on dementia might most fruitfully proceed in the future.

THE NATURE OF PSYCHOLOGICAL RESEARCH INTO DEMENTIA

Before passing on to more fundamental questions, some comment on the general characteristics of the research so far carried out on dementia has to be made. In particular, research on dementia has been extremely varied. In one sense this heterogeneity is not surprising and ought to be welcomed. It could merely reflect the wide range of functional disturbances that are associated with dementia, and the use of a large number of different but appropriate techniques in an attempt to find answers to the varied questions. This may be true to some extent but the heterogeneity also has some much less desirable aspects. It often reflects a situation in which there has been a relative shortage of research of the sort that follows up a particular problem with a series of interrelated experiments. There have been some exceptions, for example the work of Kendrick and of Walton and Black on diagnostic assessment, and that of Inglis and the present writer on memory. However there is a regrettably high incidence of 'one-off' investigations in which a more or less promising start has been made but not taken any further.

An important consequence of this is that the total picture of the state of knowledge relating to any aspect of the psychology of dementia, with the possible exception of memory, can only be built up by integrating information from a wide range of different investigators using different techniques and subject populations that may not be completely comparable. Although this point has not been continually brought up in previous chapters, its consequences are all pervasive and most conclusions must be considered subject to the qualifications that this situation obviously entails.

Another regrettable feature of most work on dementia is that it tends to fall into two unrelated types. There is a range of experimental and theoretical work on the psychopathology of dementia which is generally aimed at trying to understand the nature of the various behavioural deficits that occur. Most of this is of little practical consequence other than the rather general long-term possibility that a thorough understanding of the incapacities will provide a useful basis for remedial or ameliorative action. In contrast, the investigations directly concerned with clinical problems are heavily biased towards the application of psychometric tests and take very little account of the experimental findings.

Such a divorce between the theoretical and the practical is unfortunately all too common in abnormal and clinical psychology and by no means confined to dementia. In other aspects of abnormal and clinical psychology there is a tendency for this dichotomy to become less apparent. Similarly, in the case of dementia, the recent interest in possible ways of managing the demented patient and minimizing his incapacities may lead to some better coordination of effort. It may be that the clinician can start to utilize the results of fundamental research (e.g., that on conditioning), and the psychologist interested in more fundamental issues can attack problems that have a more direct bearing on the practical situation.

DEMENTIA AS ABNORMAL AGEING

The specific hypothesis that dementia constitutes an accelerated ageing of the nervous system has been dealt with in Chapter Seven. In general the approach used was to argue that if this hypothesis is correct then the changes produced by dementia must exactly match those produced by normal ageing. The literature was then examined with a view to identifying any apparently negative findings since a single, well established, negative instance would be enough to invalidate the hypothesis as an adequate explanation of dementia without the need to incorporate any other factors. It was concluded that the available evidence suffered from methodological difficulties but, on balance, there is some reason to doubt that the accelerated ageing hypothesis will suffice as a total explanation.

Regardless of whether this particular hypothesis, with its important aetiological implications, can offer a total explanation of dementia it is worthwhile considering the other side of the coin to see what parallels can be drawn between dementia and normal ageing. In particular to what extent can dementia be considered, even loosely, as an exaggeration or distortion of the normal ageing process?

At a superficial level there are numerous similarities between dementia and normal ageing. Both normal ageing and its apparently aberrant form, dementia, produce changes in a wide range of psychological functions such as intellect, memory, and personality. Many of the concepts used to describe the behaviour of demented patients were adumbrated in the brief review of the processes of normal ageing given in Chapter Two. The neuropathological and neurophysiological changes associated with dementia also bear considerable similarity to the developments in corresponding systems observed during normal ageing.

When the psychological findings in normal ageing and dementia are compared in greater detail the position looks much more ambiguous. In the case of intellectual changes the same explanatory notions have been used, e.g. a loss of fluid rather than crystallized intelligence. On the other hand, despite the proliferation of explanatory ideas of this kind, none of them has been shown to be unequivocally applicable to either normal or abnormal ageing. Similar comments can be made about the changes in memory. Both in dementia and normal ageing there is evidence of a difficulty in the acquisition of new information and for both there is also some evidence which could be interpreted as implicating retrieval processes. To take the question any further it would be necessary to use directly comparable experimental techniques to examine both the changes produced by normal ageing and the effects of dementia. Unfortunately this has yet to be done.

The notion of dementia as abnormal ageing in the sense of simply being normal ageing writ large has many attractions as a convenient summary of most of the known consequences of dementia. Following the discussion in Chapter Seven, it is more likely than not that this is not an entirely accurate description of dementia. In the present state of knowledge it is difficult to gauge just how accurate it is.

POSSIBLE FUTURE TRENDS

It is always extremely difficult to predict where future work will lead whatever the area of study. It could also be argued that almost the only thing that prognostications about future trends have in common is that they are almost always ultimately proved wrong. All that can be done is to try to point out the directions in which future work is most likely to lead to worthwhile additions to knowledge and developments in clinical practice. In recent years the most consistent trend in clinical psychology as a whole has been to reject the psychologist's more traditional role of evaluation and assessment, and to emphasize the active intervention in patients' problems using psychological techniques to modify behaviour in the desired direction.

Psychological endeavour with all types of patients who have organic disorder of the brain has lagged behind in these matters, and there is till a strong commitment to the role of assessment with comparatively little attention being devoted to therapy and management. This is aptly illustrated by a recent volume which purports to present current trends in work with brain-damaged populations (Reitan and Davison, 1974). Reitan and Davison's book is almost entirely devoted to the question of assessment, and the possible amelioration of behavioural deficits merits only the occasional sentence or brief comment. The same is also still very much the case in the particular instance of dementia. In preparing Chapter 8, which dealt with assessment, the writer was very much aware of a need to be selective in order to cut a vast and often repetitive literature down to size. In the following chapter the reverse was true. Whilst there are enough preliminary studies of psychological approaches to management to indicate the likelihood of being able to influence the behaviour of demented patients by psychological and social means, there is an acute shortage of information to show which specific procedures are likely to be of most use in attaining certain goals.

It is therefore being argued that the most obvious and desirable future direction that psychological endeavour can take in this field is towards greater involvement in the management and amelioration of the condition. As we have seen in Chapter Nine, a modest start has been made in this direction but there are reasons why the present might be an appropriate time to make a major commitment to this.

Firstly, it is known that demented patients may survive for a considerable number of years after the onset of the illness and even after later admission to hospital as a long-stay patient (Shah *et al.*, 1969). The general tendency, in practice if not in professed intent, is to 'write them off' once the diagnosis has been made. This is reprehensible on humanitarian grounds unless all possible ways of improving the quality of life have been shown to be failures. Another reason is the recent medical interest in ways of halting or even reversing the processes that underlie dementia. So far there have been no really impressive breakthroughs but the situation is not without promise. It is appropriate that the search for ways to halt the physical progress of the disease should be matched by complementary research into methods to modify and to compensate for psychological deficits.

Finally techniques have been devised which can favourably modify the behaviour of other types of patient with severe psychological handicaps. Possibly the best example in this context is the use of operant techniques with the severely retarded. Such techniques deserve at least an extensive trial with the demented.

Although there are also some important points of difference, an interesting parallel can be drawn between the situation with regard to dementia at the present time and that which has existed in the past in the field of mental retardation. As Clarke and Clarke (1974) illustrate, it is only necessary to go back a quarter of a century to find even well known and highly respected textbooks on mental retardation which gave an extremely pessimistic view of the capabilities and potential of the severely mentally retarded. Following the work of a small number of pioneers it has become increasingly widely accepted that the all too recent pessimism was grossly exaggerated, and the severely retarded have been found to be capable of far more than was ever imagined. All that was required was the development of appropriate training techniques and the confidence to put them into effect. The earlier successes have attracted greater interest in the management of mental retardation with a consequent rapid expansion in knowledge and practice.

In the case of dementia we are still largely in the era of profound pessimism although knowledge about the basic psychological processes in dementia is slowly accumulating. The time now seems ripe to establish finally that the previous therapeutic nihilism is unfounded. Whilst there are also obvious significant differences between the problems of mental retardation and dementia (e.g., the fact that dementia inevitably involves a slow deterioration) the recent history of mental retardation warns us that the realms of possibility may be wider than we would ever expect.

Whilst the problem of management provides the area most in need of extensive development, and is probably the most likely to yield a valuable pay off, this does not mean that other aspects of the psychology of dementia are not worthy of continuing attention. This writer does not foresee any major breakthrough in techniques of assessment although some attention could usefully be given to a number of specific points.

One of these is the limitation to the efficiency of diagnostic tests caused by those depressed patients who give scores on learning tests that are down to the level of demented subjects. It is possible that depressed patients do badly not because of an actual impairment in memory but because of other factors. Knowledge of the reasons why they fail on tasks could lead to means for detecting such cases and not erroneously classifying them as demented. Several possibilities could be suggested. Some depressed patients may be so preoccupied with their own gloomy concerns that they fail to attend adequately, or when depressed some people may adopt very conservative response strategies. They may then fail to give the desired response because they are not sure enough in their own minds that it is correct. In Southampton, Lewis and the present writer have made a preliminary, and as yet unpublished, investigation of this latter possibility by using a memory task which permitted an analysis in terms of signal detection theory. The results seem to suggest that depressed patients discriminate between the to-be-remembered stimuli and the new stimuli as well as normal control subjects and very much better than those with dementia. However the total number of correct identifications appears to be reduced in the depressed group as compared with the normal controls because of the use of a much more conservative response criterion.

Other potentially useful developments in assessment have been mentioned in Chapter 8. The work on automated testing needs to be followed through systematically. Nott and Fleminger's (1975) demonstration of the low reliability in the initial diagnosis of dementia means that the commonly used tests should be subjected to further validation. Ideally this should be done by applying the test to a random sample of cases, referred because of the need to make a differential diagnosis between dementia and depression with the diagnosis being confirmed by long-term follow-up of the cases used.

In the case of more fundamental research the regrettable divorce between theory and practice has already been commented upon. There is a pressing need to understand more fully those processes that could underlie practical attempts to improve the functioning of demented patients. Examples of topics that could relate to clinical applications are conditioning and learning, the factors that influence social behaviour in the demented (because the level of social interaction is likely to be an important determinant of the quality of life), and even such basic points as the relation between sensory and behavioural deficits. If sensory deficits are related to senile behavioural deterioration, as has recently been claimed by O'Neil and Calhoun (1975), this has an important though simple implication for clinical practice in indicating the need for each individual to be carefully evaluated with regard to the provision of sensory prostheses.

At a more purely theoretical level further opportunities for future work arise from the fact that the processes discussed in Chapter 5 are as yet poorly investigated in dementia. In addition the work on intellectual changes has a distinctly old fashioned air and this problem needs to be exposed to more modern techniques. Although memory loss is the most satisfactorily investigated area the developments are lagging a little behind current thinking in the field of normal memory. Research so far has been dominated by structural models of memory which invoke two or more separate memory stores (e.g., short- and long-term memory). Modern theorizing about normal memory is increasingly abandoning this kind of model for an approach which emphasizes coding and levels of processing (see Craik and Lockhart, 1972, for a seminal paper on this issue). The two types of model are not necessarily incompatible but the change represents a considerable shift in emphasis, and the nature of the memory defect in dementia needs to be re-examined with the newer theoretical constructs in mind.

FINAL COMMENT

It is hoped that this book will have illustrated that the topic of dementia does have a 'changing perspective' (Alexander, 1972) and that some worthwhile progress has been made both in understanding the nature of the condition and in finding ways of ameliorating its effects. Nevertheless, as the preceding section implies, dementia is still a relatively undeveloped field as far as psychology is concerned. It also presents the psychologists with a number of stimulating challenges. Despite the undeniably unattractive image that dementia still has, the problems that it presents are as inherently worthwhile and interesting as those connected with any other branch of applied psychology. It is felt that this book will have been justified if other psychologists are inspired to look at dementia rather more closely than is usually the case.

References

Abrahams, J. P., and Birren, J. E. (1973). Reaction time as a function of age and behavioral predisposition to coronary heart disease. *J. Geront.*, **28**, 471–478.

Acklesberg, S. B. (1944). Vocabulary and mental deterioration in senile dementia. *J. abnorm. soc. Psychol.*, **39**, 393–406.

Adams, R. D., Fisher, C. M., Hakim, S., Ojemann, R. G., and Sweet, W. H. (1965). Symptomatic occult hydrocephalus with 'normal' cerebrospinal fluid pressure: a treatable syndrome. *New Engl. J. Med.*, **273**, 117–126.

Ajuriaguerra, J. de., Richard, J., Rodriguez, R., and Tissot, R. (1966). Quelques aspects de la désintégration des praxies ideomotrices dans les démences du grand âge. *Cortex*, **2**, 434–462.

Ajuriaguerra, J. de., Strejilevitch, M., and Tissot, R. (1963). A propos de quelques conduites devant le miroir de sujets atteints de syndromes démentiels du grand age. *Neuropsychologia*, **1**, 59–73.

Alexander, D. A. (1970). Some tests of intelligence and learning for elderly psychiatric patients: a validation study. *Br. J. soc. clin. Psychol.*, **12**, 188–193.

Alexander, D. A. (1972). 'Senile dementia': a changing perspective. *Br. J. Psychiat.*, **121**, 207–214.

Ames, L. B., Learned, J., Metraux, R. W., and Walker, R. N. (1954). *Rorschach Responses in Old Age*. Hoeber-Harper, New York.

Aminoff, M. J., Marshall, J., Smith, E. M., and Wyke, M. (1975). Pattern of intellectual impairment in Huntington's chorea. *Psychol. Med.*, **5**, 169–172.

Amster, L. B., and Krauss, J. (1974). The relationship between life crises and mental deterioration in old age. *Int. J. Aging Hum. Devel.*, **5**, 51–55.

Ankus, M. (1970). Investigation of operant behavior in elderly psychiatric patients with memory disorder. Unpublished Ph.D. Thesis, York University, Ontario.

Ankus, M., and Quarrington, B. (1972). Operant behavior in the memory disordered. *J. Geront.*, **27**, 500–510.

Averbach, E., and Coriell, A. S. (1961). Short-term memory in vision. *Bell Syst. Tech. J.*, **40**, 309–328.

Baddeley, A. D. (1966a). Short-term memory for word sequences as a function of acoustic, semantic and formal similarity. *Quart. J. exp. Psychol.*, **18**, 362–365.

Baddeley, A. D. (1966b). The influence of acoustic and semantic similarity on long-term memory for word sequences. *Quart. J. exp. Psychol.*, **18**, 302–309.

Baddeley, A. D., and Dale, H. C. A. (1966). The effect of semantic similarity on retroactive interference in long- and short-term memory. *J. verb. Learn. verb. Behav.*, **5**, 417–420.

Ball, J. A. C., and Taylor, A. R. (1967). Effects of cyclandelate on mental function and cerebral blood flow in elderly patients. *Br. Med. J.*, **3**, 525–528.

Barker, M. G., and Lawson, J. S. (1968). Nominal aphasia in dementia. *Br. J. Psychiat.*, **114**, 1351–1356.

Barnes, J. A. (1974). Effects of reality orientation classroom on memory loss, confusion and disorientation in geriatric patients. *Gerontologist*, **14**, 138–142.

Barns, E. K., Sack, A., and Shore, H. (1973). Guidelines to treatment approaches: modalities and methods for use with the aged. *Gerontologist*, **13**, 513–527.

Bartlett, F. C. (1932). *Remembering*. Cambridge University Press, Cambridge.

Baumeister, A. A. (1967). Problems in comparative studies of mental retardates and normals. *Amer. J. Ment. Defic.*, **71**, 869–875.

Belbin, E. (1958). Methods of training older workers. *Ergonomics*, **1**, 207–221.

Belbin, E., and Downs, S. (1964). Activity learning and the older worker. *Ergonomics*, **7**, 429–438.

Bender, A. D., Kormendy, C. G., and Powell, R. (1970). Pharmacological control of aging. *Exp. Geront.*, **5**, 97–129.

Bender, L. (1946). *Instructions for the Use of the Visual Motor Gestalt Test*. American Orthopsychiatric Association, New York.

Benson, D. F. (1974). Normal pressure hydrocephalus: a controversial entity. *Geriatrics*, **29**, 125–132.

Benton, A. L. (1963). *The Revised Visual Retention Test*. State University of Iowa, Iowa City.

Bergmann, K. (1969). The epidemiology of senile dementia. *Br. J. Hosp. Med.*, **2**, 727–732.

Bevans, H. G. (1972). Development of experimental method assessing attention, learning and recall in geriatric patients. In H. M. van Praag and A. F. Kalverboer (Eds) *Ageing of the Central Nervous System: Biological and Psychological Aspects*. De Erven F. Bohn, Haarlem.

Birren, J. E. (1964). *The Psychology of Aging*. Prentice-Hall, New Jersey.

Birren, J. E., and Botwinick, J. (1951). The relation of writing speed to age and to the senile psychoses. *J. consult. Psychol.*, **15**, 243–249.

Birren, J. E., and Botwinick, J. (1955). Age differences in finger, jaw, and foot reaction time to auditory stimuli. *J. Geront.*, **10**, 429–432.

Blessed, G., Tomlinson, B. E., and Roth, M. (1968). The association between quantitative measures of dementia and of senile change in the cerebral grey matter of elderly subjects. *Br. J. Psychiat.*, **114**, 797–811.

Bolton, N. (1967). A psychometric investigation of the psychiatric syndromes of old age: measures of intelligence, learning, memory, extraversion and neuroticism. Unpublished Ph.D. Thesis. University of Newcastle-upon-Tyne.

Bolton, N., Britton, P. G., and Savage, R. D. (1966). Some normative data on the WAIS and its indices in an aged population. *J. clin. Psychol.*, **22**, 184–188.

Bolton, N., Savage, R. D., and Roth, M. (1967). The Modified Word Learning Test and the aged psychiatric patient. *Br. J. Psychiat.*, **113**, 1139–1140.

Botwinick, J. (1966). Cautiousness with advanced age. *J. Geront.*, **21**, 347–353.

Botwinick, J. (1971). Sensory set factors in age differences in reaction time. *J. Gen. Psychol.*, **119**, 241–249.

Botwinick, J. (1973). *Aging and Behavior*. Springer, New York.

Botwinick, J., and Birren, J. E. (1951a). The measurement of intellectual decline in the senile psychoses. *J. consult. Psychol.*, **15**, 145–150.

Botwinick, J., and Birren, J. E. (1951b). Differential decline in the Wechsler–Bellevue subtests in the senile psychoses. *J. Geront.*, **6**, 365–368.

Botwinick, J., Brinley, J. F., and Birren, J. E. (1957). Set in relation to age. *J. Geront.*, **12**, 300–305.

Botwinick, J., Brinley, J. F., and Birren, J. E. (1958). The effect of motivation by electric shocks on reaction time in relation to age. *Amer. J. Psychol.*, **71**, 408–411.

Botwinick, J., and Kornetsky, C. (1960). Age differences in the acquisition and extinction of GSR. *J. Geront.*, **15**, 83–84.

Botwinick, J., and Thompson, L. W. (1966). Components of reaction time in relation to age and sex. *J. Gen. Psychol.*, **108**, 175–183.

Bouvier, J. B., Passeron, O., and Chupin, M. P. (1974). Psychometric study of praxilene. *J. Internat. Med. Rs.*, **2**, 59–65.

Bower, H. M. (1967). Sensory stimulation and the treatment of senile dementia. *Med. J. Aust.*, **1**, 1113–1119.

Bowers, M. B., Anderson, G. K., Blomeier, E. C., and Pelz K. (1967). Brain syndrome and behavior in geriatric remotivation groups. *J. Geront.*, **22**, 348–352.

Boyarsky, R. E., and Eisdorfer, C. (1972). Forgetting in older persons. *J. Geront.*, **27**, 254–258.

Boyd, D. A. (1936). A contribution to the psychopathology of Alzheimer's disease. *Amer. J. Psychiat.*, **93**, 155–175.

Brain, W. R., and Walton, J. N. (1969). *Brain's Diseases of the Nervous System*. Oxford University Press, London.

Braun, H. W., and Geiselhart, R. (1959). Age differences in the acquisition and extinction of the conditioned eyelid response. *J. Exp. Psychol.*, **57**, 386–388.

Brilliant, P. J., and Gynther, M. D. (1963). Relationship between performance on three tests for organicity and selected patient variables. *J. consult. Psychol.*, **27**, 474–479.

Britton, A., Bernstein, L. L., Brunse, A. J., Buttiglien, M. W., Cherlein, A., McCormack, J. H., and Lewis, D. J. (1972). Failure of ingestion of RNA to enhance human learning. *J. Geront.*, **27**, 478–481.

Broadbent, D. E. (1954). The role of auditory localization in attention and memory span. *J. Exp. Psychol.*, **47**, 191–196.

Broadbent, D. E. (1958). *Perception and Communication*. Pergamon Press, Oxford.

Broadbent, D. E. (1970). Psychological aspects of short-term and long-term memory. *Proc. R. Soc. Lond.*, **175**, 333–350.

Broadbent, D. E. (1971). *Decision and Stress*. Academic Press, London.

Brody, E. M., Kleban, M. H., Lawton, M. P., and Moss, M. (1974). Longitudinal look at excess disabilities in the mentally impaired aged. *J. Geront.*, **29**, 79–84.

Brody, E. M., Kleban, M. H., Lawton, M. P., and Silverman, H. A. (1971). Excess disabilities of mentally impaired aged: impact of individualized treatment. *Gerontologist*, **11**, 124–132.

Brody, M. B. (1942). A psychometric study of dementia. *J. Ment. Sci.*, **88**, 512–533.

Bromley, D. B. (1972). Intellectual changes in adult life and old age: a commentary on the assumptions underlying the study of intelligence. In H. M. van Praag and A. F. Kalverboer (Eds) *Aging of the Central Nervous System: Biological and Psychological Aspects*. De Erven F. Bohn, Haarlem.

Bromley, D. B. (1974). *The Psychology of Human Ageing*. 2nd ed., Penguin, Harmondsworth.

Brook, P., Gegun, G., and Mather, M. (1975). Reality orientation, a therapy for psychogeriatric patients: a controlled study. *Br. J. Psychiat.*, **127**, 42–45.

Brosin, H. W. (1952). Contributions of psychoanalysis to the study of organic cerebral disorders. In F. Alexander and H. Rees (Eds) *Dynamic Psychiatry*. University of Chicago Press, Chicago.

Brown, C. C., Gantt, W. H., and Whitman, J. R. (1960). Measures of adaptability in senility. In P. H. Hoch and J. Zubin (Eds) *Psychopothology of Aging*. The American Psychopathological Association, New York.

Brozeck, J. (1955). Personality changes with age: an item analysis of the Minnesota Multiphasic Personality Inventory. *J. Geront.*, **10**, 194–206.

Bruner, J. S., Goodnow, J. J., and Austin, G. A. (1956). *A Study of Thinking*. Wiley, New York.

Bull, J. W. D. (1961). The volume of the cerebral ventricles. *Neurology*, **11**, 1–13.

Burhenne, H. J., and Davies, H. (1963). The ventricular span in cerebral pneumography. *Amer. J. Roentgenol.*, **90**, 1176–1181.

Busse, E. W. (1969). Theories of aging. In E. W. Busse and E. Pfeiffer (Eds) *Behavior and Adaptation in Late Life*. Little, Brown & Co., Boston.

Butters, N., and Cermak, L. S. (1974). Some comments on Warrington and Baddeley's report of normal short-term memory in amnesic patients. *Neuropsychologia*, **12**, 283–285.

Caird, W. K. (1966). Memory loss in the senile psychoses: organic or psychogenic. *Psychol. Rep.*, **18**, 788–790.

Caird, W. K., and Hannah, F. (1964). Short-term memory disorder in elderly psychiatric patients. *Dis. nerv. Syst.*, **25**, 564–568.

Caird, W. K., and Inglis, J. (1961). The short-term storage of auditory and visual two-channel digits by elderly patients with memory disorder. *J. Ment. Sci.*, **107**, 1062–1069.

Caird, W. K., Laverty, S. G., and Inglis, J. (1963), Sedation and sleep thresholds in elderly patients with memory disorder. *Geront. Clin.*, **5**, 55–62.

Caird, W. K., Sanderson, R. E., and Inglis, J. (1962). Cross validation of a learning test for use with elderly psychiatric patients. *J. Ment. Sci.*, **108**, 368–370.

Cameron, D. E. (1940). Certain aspects of defects of recent memory occurring in psychoses of the senium. *Arch. Neurol. Psychiat.*, **43**, 987–992.

Cameron, D. E. (1941). Studies in senile nocturnal delirium. *Psychiat. Quart.*, **15**, 47–53.

Cameron, D. E. (1958). The use of nucleic acid in aging patients with memory impairment. *Amer. J. Psychiat.*, **114**, 943.

Cameron, D. E., and Solyom, L. (1961). Effects of ribonucleic acid on memory. *Geriatrics*, **16**, 74–81.

Cameron, D. E., Sved, S., Solyom, L., Wainrib, B., and Baric, H. (1963). Effects of ribonucleic acid on memory defects in the aged. *Amer. J. Psychiat.*, **120**, 320–325.

Cameron, N. (1938). A study of thinking in senile deterioration and schizophrenic disorganisation. *Amer. J. Psychol.*, **51**, 650–664.

Canter, A., and Straumanis, J. J. (1969). Performance of senile and healthy aged persons on the Bender test. *Percept. Motor Skills*, **28**, 695–698.

Cattell, R. B. (1943). The measurement of adult intelligence. *Psychol. Bull.*, **3**, 153–193.

Cattell, R. B. (1965). *The Scientific Analysis of Personality*. Penguin, Harmondsworth.

Cermak, L. S., Butters, N., and Goodglass, H. (1971). The extent of memory loss in Korsakoff patients. *Neuropsychologia*, **9**, 307–315.

Chown, S. M. (1960). A factor analysis of the Wesley Rigidity Inventory: its relationship to age and non-verbal intelligence. *J. abnorm. soc. Psychol.*, **61**, 491–494.

Chown, S. M. (1962). Rigidity and age. In C. Tibbitts and W. Donahue (Eds) *Social and Psychological Aspects of Aging*. Columbia University Press, New York.

Clarke, A. M., and Clarke, A. D. B. (1973). Mental Subnormality. In H. J. Eysenck (Ed.) *Handbook of Abnormal Psychology*. 2nd ed., Pitman, London.

Clarke, A. M., and Clarke, A. D. B. (1974). Severe subnormality: capacity and performance. In A. M. Clarke and A. D. B. Clarke (Eds) *Mental Deficiency: The Changing Outlook*. 3rd ed., Methuen, London.

Clark, L. E., and Knowles, J. B. (1973). Age differences in dichotic listening performance. *J. Geront.*, **28**, 173–178.

Cleveland, S., and Dysinger, D. (1944). Mental deterioration in senile psychosis. *J. abnorm. soc. Psychol.*, **39**, 368–372.

Coltheart, M. (1972). Visual information processing. In P. C. Dodwell (Ed.) *New Horizons in Psychology*. 2nd ed., Penguin, Harmondsworth.

Comfort, A. (1973). Theories of aging. In J. C. Brocklehurst (Ed.) *Textbook of Geriatric Medicine*. Churchill and Livingstone, Edinburgh.

Corsellis, J. A. N. (1962). *Mental Illness and the Ageing Brain*. Oxford University Press, London.

Corsellis, J. A. N. (1970). The limbic areas in Alzheimer's disease and related conditions associated with dementia. In G. Wolstenholme and M. O'Connor (Eds) *Alzheimer's Disease*. Churchill, London.

Cosin, L. Z., Mort, M., Post, F., Westrop, C., and Williams, M. (1958). Experimental treatment of persistent senile confusion. *Internat. J. soc. Psychiat.*, **4**, 24–42.

Costello, C. G. (1970). *Symptoms of Psychopathology*, Wiley, New York.

Cox, J. R., and Orme, J. E. (1973). Body water, electrolytes and psychological test performance in elderly patients. *Geront. Clin.*, **15**, 203–208.

Craik, F. I. M. (1968). Short-term memory and the aging process. In G. A. Talland (Ed.) *Human Aging and Behavior*, Academic Press, New York.

Craik, F. I. M., and Lockhart, R. S. (1972). Levels of processing: a framework for memory research. *J. verb. Learn. verb. Behav.*, **11**, 671–684.

Critchley, M. (1933). Discussion on the mental and physical symptoms of the presenile dementias. *Proc. R. Soc. Med.*, **26**, 1077–1084.

Critchley, M. (1964). The neurology of psychotic speech. *Br. J. Psychiat.*, **110**, 353–364.

Crookes, T. G. (1974). Indices of early dementia on the WAIS. *Psychol. Rep.*, **34**, 374.

Crookes, T. G. and McDonald, K. G. (1972). Benton's Visual Retention Test in the differentiation of depression and early dementia. *Br. J. soc. clin. Psychol.*, **11**, 66–69.

Cumming, E., and Henry, W. (1961). *Growing Old: The Process of Disengagement.* Basic Books, New York.

Cunningham, W. R., Clayton, V., and Overton, W. (1975). Fluid and crystallized intelligence in young adulthood and old age. *J. Geront.*, **30**, 53–55.

Dayan, A. D. (1971). Presenile dementia: some pathological problems and possibilities. *Proc. R. Soc. Med.*, **64**, 829–831.

De Renzi, E., and Vignolo, L. A. (1962). The token test: a sensitive test to detect receptive disturbances in aphasias. *Brain*, **85**, 665–678.

Desai, M. (1952). The test-retest reliability on the Progressive Matrices Test. *Br. J. med. Psychol.*, **25**, 48–53.

Dixon, J. C. (1965). Cognitive structure in senile conditions with some suggestions for developing a brief screening test of mental status. *J. Geront.*, **20**, 41–49.

Dorken, H. (1954). Psychometric differences between senile dementia and normal senescent decline. *Canad. J. Psychol.*, **8**, 187–194.

Dorken, H., and Greenbloom, G. C. (1953). Psychological investigations of senile dementia. II. The Wechsler–Bellevue Adult Intelligence Scale. *Geriatrics*, **8**, 324–333.

Dorken, H., and Kral, V. A. (1951). Psychological investigation of senile dementia. *Geriatrics*, **6**, 151–163.

Drachman, D. A., and Arbit, J. (1965). Memory and the hippocampal complex. *Arch. Neurol.*, **15**, 52–61.

Drachman, D. A., and Leavitt, J. (1972). Memory impairment in the aged: storage versus retrieval deficits. *J. exp. Psychol.*, **93**, 302–308.

Duffy, E. (1962). *Activation and Behavior.* Wiley, New York.

Edwards, A. E., and Vine, D. B. (1963). Personality changes with age: their dependency on concomitant intellectual decline. *J. Geront.*, **18**, 182–184.

Eichorn, O. (1965). The effect of cyclandelate on cerebral circulation. *Vascul. Dis.*, **2**, 303–315.

Engeset, A., and Lonnum, A. (1958). Third ventricles of 12 mm width or more. *Acta. Radiol.*, **50**, 5–11.

Erber, J. T. (1974). Age differences in recognition memory. *J. Geront.*, **29**, 177–189.

Ernst, B., Dalby, M. A., and Dalby, A. (1970a). Aphasic disturbances in presenile dementia. *Acta Neurol. Scand., Suppl.*, **43**, 99–100.

Ernst, B., Dalby, A., and Dalby, M. A. (1970b). Gnostic-praxic disturbances in presenile dementia. *Acta Neurol. Scand., Suppl.*, **43**, 101–102.

Eysenck, H. J. (1960). *Handbook of Abnormal Psychology.* Pitman, London.

Eysenck, M. D. (1945a). A study of certain qualitative aspects of problem solving behaviour in senile dementia patients. *J. Ment. Sci.*, **91**, 337–345.

Eysenck, M. D. (1945b). An exploratory study of mental organisation in senility. *J. neurol. Psychiat.*, **8**, 15–21.

Eysenck, M. W. (1975). Retrieval from semantic memory as a function of age. *J. Geront.*, **30**, 174–180.

Ferenczi, S. (1922). Psychoanalysis and the mental disorders of general paralysis of the insane. Reprinted in M. Balint (Ed.) *Final Contributions to the Problems and Methods of Psychoanalysis.* The Hogarth Press, London, 1955.

Ferm, L. (1974). Behavioral activities in demented geriatric patients. Study based on evaluations made by nursing staff and on patients scores on a simple psychometric test. *Geront. Clin.*, **16**, 185–194.

Fine, E. W., Lewis, D., Villa-Landa, I., and Blakemore, C. B. (1970). The effect of cyclandelate on mental function in patients with arteriosclerotic brain disease. *Br. J. Psychiat.*, **117**, 157–161.

Fisch, M., Goldfarb, A. I., Shahinian, S. P., and Turner, H. (1968). Chronic brain syndrome in the community aged. *Arch. Gen. Psychiat.*, **18**, 739–745.

Folsom, J. C. (1967). Intensive hospital therapy for geriatric patients. *Curr. Psychiat. Ther.*, **7**, 209–215.

Folsom, J. C. (1968). Reality orientation for the elderly patient. *J. Geriat. Psychiat.*, **1**, 291–307.

Freeman, T., and Gathercole, C. E. (1966). Perseveration—the clinical symptoms—in chronic schizophrenia and organic dementia. *Br. J. Psychiat.*, **112**, 27–32.

Gailliard, J. M. (1970). La désintégration du schéma corporel dans les états démentiels du grand age. *J. Psychol. Norm. Pathol.*, **67**, 443–472.

Gantt, W. H. (1950). The conditioned reflex as an aid in the study of the psychiatric patient. In P. H. Hock and J. Zubin (Eds) *Relation of Psychological Tests to Psychiatry*. Grune and Stratton, New York.

Ganzler, H. (1964). Motivation as a factor in the psychological deficit of aging. *J. Geront.*, **19**, 425–429.

Garside, R. F., Kay, D. W. K., and Roth, M. (1965). Old age mental disorders in Newcastle-upon-Tyne. Part III. A factorial study of medical, psychiatric and social characteristics. *Br. J. Psychiat.*, **111**, 939–946.

Gathercole, C. E. (1968). *Assessment in Clinical Psychology*. Penguin, Harmondsworth.

Gedye, J. L., Exton-Smith, A. N., and Wedgwood, J. (1972). A method of measuring mental performance in the elderly and its use in a pilot clinical trial of medofexonate in organic dementi. *Age and Ageing*, **1**, 74–80.

Gedye, J. L., and Miller, E. (1969). The automation of psychological assessment. *Internat. J. Man-Machine Stud.*, **1**, 237–262.

Gedye, J. L., and Miller, E. (1970). Developments in automated testing systems. In P. J. Mittler (Ed.) *The Psychological Assessment of Mental and Physical. Handicap*. Methuen, London.

Gerboth, R. (1950). A study of the two forms of the Wechsler–Bellevue Intelligence Scale. *J. Consult. Psychol.*, **15**, 365–370.

Gilbert, J. G., and Levee, R. F. (1971). Patterns of declining memory. *J. Geront.*, **26**, 70–75.

Gilmore, A. J. J. (1972). Personality in the elderly: problems of methodology. *Age and Ageing*, **1**, 227–232.

Glaister, B. R. (1971). An ordinate comparison method of calculating brain damage probability. *Br. J. soc. clin. Psychol.*, **10**, 367–374.

Glanzer, M., and Cunitz, A. R. (1966). Two storage mechanisms in free recall. *J. verb. Learn. verb. Behav.*, **5**, 351–360.

Goldfarb, A. I., Hochstadt, N. J., Jacobson, J. H., and Weinstein, E. A. (1972). Hyperbaric oxygen treatment of organic mental syndrome in aged persons. *J. Geront.*, **27**, 212–217.

Goldstein, K., and Scheerer, M. (1941). Abstract and concrete behavior: an experimental study with special tests. *Psychol. Monogr.*, **53**, No. 2.

Gonen, J. Y., and Brown, L. (1968). Role of vocabulary in deterioration and restitution of mental functioning. *Proc. Ann. Congr. A. P. A.*, p. 469.

Gordon, E. B. (1968). Serial EEG studies in presenile dementia. *Br. J. Psychiat.*, **114**, 779–780.

Gordon, S. K., and Clark, W. W. (1974). Application of signal detection theory to prose recall and recognition in elderly and young adults. *J. Geront.*, **29**, 64–72.

Gosling, R. H. (1955). The association of dementia with radiologically demonstrated cerebral atrophy. *J. neurol. neurosurg. Psychiat.*, **18**, 129–133.

Gottfries, C. G., Gottfries, I., and Roos, B. E. (1970). Homvanillic acid and 5-hydroxy-indoleacetic acid in cerebrospinal fluid related to rated mental and motor impairment in senile and presenile dementia. *Acta Psychiat. Scand.*, **46**, 99–105.

Goulet, L. R., and Baltes, P. B. (1970). *Life-Span Developmental Psychology.* Academic Press, New York.

Graham, F. K., and Kendall, B. S. (1960). *Memory-for-Designs Test: Revised General Manual.* Percept. Motor Skills Monogr. Suppl. No. 11.

Gruneberg, M. (1970). A dichotomous theory of memory—unproven or unprovable? *Acta Psychol.*, **34**, 489–496.

Grünthal, E. (1926). Über die Alzheimersche Krankheit. *Ztschr. f. d. ges. Neurol. u. Psychiat.*, **101**, 128–146.

Guertin, W. H., Rabin, A. L., Frank, G. H., and Ladd, C. E. (1962). Research on the Wechsler Intelligence Scale for Adults, 1955–1966. *Psychol. Bull.*, **59**, 1–26.

Gustafson, L., and Hagberg, B. (1975). Dementia with onset in the presenile period: a cross sectional study. *Acta. Psychiat. Scand.*, Suppl. No. 257.

Gustafson, L., and Risberg, J. (1974). Regional cerebral blood flow related to psychiatric symptoms in dementia with onset in the presenile period. *Acta Psychiat. Scand.*, **50**, 516–538.

Hain, J. D. (1964). The Bender–Gestalt Test—a scoring method for identifying brain damage. *J. consult. Psychol.*, **28**, 34–40.

Hakim, S., and Adams, R. D. (1965). The special clinical problems of symptomatic hydrocephalus with normal cerebrospinal fluid pressure. Observation on cerebrospinal dynamics. *J. Neurol. Sci.*, **2**, 307–327.

Hall, E. H., Savage, R. D., Bolton, N., Pidwell, D. M., and Blessed, G. (1972). Intellect, mental illness, and survival in the aged. *J. Geront.*, **27**, 237–244.

Hall, J. C. (1957). Reliability (internal consistency) of the Wechsler Memory Scale and correlation with the Wechsler–Bellevue Intelligence Scale. *J. consult. Psychol.*, **21**, 131–135.

Halstead, H. (1943). A psychometric study of senility. *J. Ment. Sci.*, **89**, 863–873.

Hamister, R. C. (1949). Test–re-test reliability of the Wechsler–Bellevue. *J. consult. Psychol.*, **13**, 39–43.

Hardyck, C. D. (1964). Sex differences in personality changes with age. *J. Geront.*, **19**, 78–82.

Harrell, T. W., and Harrell, M. S. (1945). Army General Classification Test scores for civilian populations. *Educ. Psychol. Meas.*, **5**, 229–239.

Hart, B., and Spearman, C. (1914). Mental tests of dementia. *J. abnorm. Psychol.*, **9**, 217–264.

Havighurst, R. J., Neugarten, B. L., and Tobin, S. S. (1968). Disengagement and patterns of aging. In B. L. Neugarten (Ed.) *Middle Age and Aging: A Reader in Psychology.* University of Chicago Press, Chicago.

Hebb, D. O. (1949). *The Organization of Behavior.* Wiley, New York.

Hedlund, S., Kohler, V., Nylin, G., Olsen, R., Rignstrom, O., Rothstrom, E., and Astrum, A. E. (1964). Cerebral blood circulation in dementia. *Acta Psychiat. Scand.*, **40**, 77–106.

Hemsi, L. K., Whitehead, A., and Post, F. (1968). Cognitive functioning and cerebral arousal in elderly depressives and dements. *J. Psychosom. Res.*, **12**, 145–156.

Hewson, L. R. (1949). The Wechsler–Bellevue Scale and the substitution test as aids in neuropsychiatric diagnosis. *J. nerv. ment. Dis.*, **109**, 158–183.

Hibbard, T. R., Migliaccio, J. N., Goldstone, S., and Lhamon, W. T. (1975). Temporal information processing by young and senior adults and patients with senile dementia. *J. Geront.*, **30**, 326–330.

Hill, D., and Driver, M. V. (1962). Electroencephalography. In Lord Brain (Ed.) *Recent Advances in Neurology and Neuropsychiatry.* Churchill, London.

Hopkins, B., and Post, F. (1955). The significance of abstract and concrete behavior in elderly psychiatric patients and control subjects. *J. Ment. Sci.*, **101**, 841–850.

Hopkins, B., and Roth, M. (1953). Psychological test performance in patients over sixty.

152

II. paraphrenics, arteriosclerotic psychosis and acute confusion. *J. Ment. Sci.*, **99**, 451–463.

Howes, D. (1964). Application of the word frequency concept to aphasia. In A. V. S. Reuck and M. O'Connor (Eds) *Ciba Foundation Symposium on Disorders of Language.* Churchill, London.

Hoyer, W. J. (1973). Application of operant techniques to the modification of elderly behavior. *Gerontologist*, **13**, 18–22.

Hoyer, W. J., Kafer, R. A., Simpson, S. C., and Hoyer, F. W. (1974). Reinstatement of verbal behavior in elderly patients using operant procedures. *Gerontologist*, **14**, 149–152.

Husen, T. (1951). The influence of schooling upon IQ. *Theoria*, **17**, 61–88.

Hydén, H. (1955). Nucleic acid and protein. In K. Elliott and A. Caldwell (Eds) *Neurochemistry: the Chemistry Dynamics of Brain and Nerves.* C. C. Thomas, Springfield, Ill.

Hydén, H. (1970). The question of a molecular basis for the memory trace. In K. H. Pribram and D. E. Broadbent (Eds) *Biology of Memory.* Academic Press, New York.

Inglis, J. (1957). An experimental study of learning and 'memory function' in elderly psychiatric patients. *J. Ment. Sci.*, **103**, 796–803.

Inglis, J. (1959a). Learning, retention and conceptual usage in elderly patients with memory disorder. *J. abnorm. soc. Psychol.*, **59**, 210–215.

Inglis, J. (1959b). A paired associate learning test for use with elderly psychiatric patients. *J. Ment. Sci.*, **105**, 440–448.

Inglis, J. (1960). Dichotic stimulation and memory disorder. *Nature*, **186**, 181–182.

Inglis, J. (1962). Psychological practice in geriatric problems. *J. Ment. Sci.*, **108**, 669–674.

Inglis, J. (1965). Immediate memory, age and brain function. In A. T. Welford and J. E. Birren (Eds) *Behavior, Aging and the Nervous System.* C. C. Thomas, Springfield, Ill.

Inglis, J. (1970). Memory disorder. In C. G. Costello (Ed.) *Symptoms of Psychopathology.* Wiley, New York.

Inglis, J. and Sanderson, R. F. (1961). Successive response to simulatneous stimulation in elderly patients with memory disorder. *J. abnorm. soc. Psychol.*, **62**, 709–712.

Inglis, J., Sykes, D. H., and Ankus, M. N. (1968). Age differences in short-term memory. In S. M. Chown and K. F. Riegel (Eds) *Psychological Functioning in Normal Aging and Senile Aged.* S. Karger, Basel.

Jacobs, E. A., Winter, P. M., Alvis, H. J., and Small, S. M. (1969). Hyperoxygenation effect on cognitive functioning in the aged. *New Engl. Med. J.*, **281**, 753–757.

Jarvik, L. F., and Falek, A. (1963). Intellectual stability and survival in the aged. *J. Geront.*, **18**, 173–176.

Judge, T. G., Urquhart, A., and Blakemore, C. B. (1973). Cyclandelate and mental functions: a double blind cross-over trial in normal elderly subjects. *Age and Ageing*, **2**, 121–124.

Katz, L., Neal, M. W., and Simon, A. (1960). Observations of psychic mechanisms in organic psychoses of the aged. In P. H. Hoch and J. Zubin (Eds) *Psychopathology of Aging.* Proc. Amer. Psychopath. Ass., New York.

Kay, D. W. K. (1962). Outcome and cause of death in mental disorders of old age: a long-term follow-up of functional and organic psychoses. *Acta Psychiat. Scand.*, **38**, 249–276.

Kay, D. W. K., Beamish, P., and Roth, M. (1964a). Old age mental disorders in Newcastle-upon-Tyne. I. A. study of prevalence. *Br. J. Psychiat.*, **110**, 146–158.

Kay, D. W. K., Beamish, P., and Roth, M. (1964b). Old age mental disorders in Newcastle-upon-Tyne. II. A study of possible social and medical causes. *Br. J. Psychiat.*, **110**, 668–682.

Kay, D. W. K., Bergmann, K., Foster, L. M., McKechnie, A. A., and Roth, M. (1970). Mental illness and hospital usage in the elderly: a random sample followed up. *Comp. Psychiat.*, **11**, 26–35.

Kazdin, A. E. (1973). Issues in behavior modification with mentally retarded persons. *Amer. J. Ment. Defic.*, **78**, 134–140.

Kazdin, A. E. (1975). *Behavior Modification in Applied Settings*. The Dorsey Press, Homewood, Ill.

Kendrick, D. C. (1965). Speed and learning in the diagnosis of diffuse brain damage in elderly subjects: a Bayesian statistical approach. *Br. J. soc. clin. Psychol.*, **4**, 141–148.

Kendrick, D. C. (1967). A cross validation study of the use of the SLT and DCT in screening for diffuse brain pathology in elderly subjects. *Br. J. med. Psychol.*, **40**, 173–178.

Kendrick, D. C. (1972). The Kendrick battery of tests; theoretical assumptions and clinical uses. *Br. J. soc. clin. Psychol.*, **4**, 63–71.

Kendrick, D. C., Parboosingh, R.-C., and Post, F. (1965). A synonym learning test for use with elderly psychiatric subjects: a validation study. *Br. J. soc. clin. Psychol.*, **4**, 63–71.

Kendrick, D. C. and Post, F. (1967). Differences in cognitive status between healthy psychiatrically ill and diffusely brain damaged elderly subjects. *Br. J. Psychiat.*, **113**, 75–81.

Kiernan, C. C. (1974). Behaviour modification. In A. M. Clarke and A. D. B. Clarke (Eds) *Mental Deficiency: The Changing Outlook*. 3rd ed., Methuen, London.

Kimble, G. A., and Pennybacker, H. S. (1963). Eyelid conditioning in young and aged subjects. *J. Genet. Psychol.*, **103**, 283–289.

Kiev, A., Chapman, L. F., Guthrie, T. C., and Wolff, H. G. (1962). The highest integrative functions and diffuse cerebral atrophy. *Neurology*, **12**, 385–393.

Kinsbourne, M. (1973). Age effect on letter span related to rate and sequential dependency. *J. Geront.*, **28**, 317–319.

Kleban, M. H., and Brody, E. M. (1972). Prediction of improvement in mentally impaired aged: personality ratings by social workers. *J. Geront.*, **27**, 69–76.

Kleban, M. H., Brody, E. M., and Lawton, M. P. (1971). Personality traits in the mentally impaired aged and their relationship to improvements in current functioning. *Gerontologist*, **11**, 134–140.

Klee, A. (1964). The relationship between clinical evaluation of mental deterioration, psychological test results and the cerebral metabolic rate of oxygen. *Acta Neurol. Scand.*, **40**, 337–345.

Kline, D. W., and Szafran, J. (1975). Age differences in backward monoptic visual noise masking. *J. Geront.*, **30**, 307–311.

Kral, V. A. (1958). Neuropsychiatric observations in an old peoples home. Studies of memory function in senescence. *J. Geront.*, **13**, 169–176.

Kral, V. A. (1962). Senescent forgetfulness: benign or malignant. *Canad. Med. Ass. J.*, **86**, 257–260.

Kral, V. A. (1966). Memory loss in the aged. *Dis. Nerv. Syst.*, **27**, 51–54.

Kral, V. A., and Durost, H. B. (1953). A comparative study of the amnesic syndrome in various organic conditions. *Amer. J. Psychiat.*, **110**, 41–47.

Larsson, T., Sjogren, T., and Jacobsen, G. (1963). Senile dementia. *Acta. Psychiat. Scand.*, Suppl. No. 167.

Laurence, M. W. (1967). Memory loss with age: a test of two strategies for its retardation. *Psychonom. Sci.*, **9**, 209–210.

Lessen, N. A., Feinberg, I., and Lane, M. H. (1960). Bilateral studies of cerebral oxygen uptake in young and aged normal subjects and in patients with organic dementia. *J. Clin. Invest.*, **39**, 491–500.

Lassen, N. A., Munck, O., and Tortey, E. R. (1957). Mental function and cerebral oxygen consumption in organic dementia. *Arch. Neurol. Psychiat.*, **77**, 126–133.

Lawson, J. S., and Barker, M. G. (1968). The assessment of nominal dysphasia in dementia. *Br. J. med. Psychol.*, **41**, 411–414.

Lawson, J. S., McGhie, A., and Chapman, J. (1967). Distractibility in schizophrenia and organic cerebral disease. *Br. J. Psychiat.*, **113**, 527–535.

Lehman, H. C. (1953). *Age and Achievement*. Oxford University Press, London.

Lehman, H. C. (1962). The most creative years of engineers and other technologists. *J. Genet. Psychol.*, **108**, 263–277.

Lehman, H. C. (1964). The relationship between chronological age and high level research output in physics and chemistry. *J. Geront.*, **19**, 157–164.

Letemendia, F., and Pampiglioni, G. (1958). Clinical and electroencephalographic observations in Alzheimer's disease. *J. neurol. neurosurg. Psychiat.*, **21**, 167–172.

Levy, R. (1969). The neurophysiology of dementia. *Br. J. Hosp. Med.*, **2**, 688–690.

Levy, R. (1972). Neurophysiological disturbances associated with psychiatric disorder in old age. In H. M. van Praag and A. F. Kalverboer (Eds) *Aging of the Central Nervous System: Biological and Psychological Aspects*. De Erven F. Bohn, Haarlem.

Levy, R., Isaacs, A., and Behrman, J. (1971). Neurophysiological correlates of senile dementia. II. The somatosensory evoked response. *Psychol. Med.*, **1**, 159–165.

Levy, R., Isaacs, A., and Hawks, G. (1970). Neurophysiological correlates of senile dementia. I. Motor and sensory nerve conduction velocity. *Psychol. Med.*, **1**, 40–47.

Levy, R., and Poole, E. W. (1966). Peripheral motor nerve conduction in elderly demented and non-demented psychiatric patients. *J. neurol. neurosurg. Psychiat.*, **29**, 362–366.

Levy, R., and Post, F. (1975). The use of an interactive computer terminal in the assessment of cognitive function in elderly psychiatric patients. *Age and Ageing*, **4**, 110–115.

Libb, J. W., and Clements, C. B. (1969). Token reinforcement in an excercise program for hospitalized geriatric patients. *Percept. Motor Skills*, **28**, 957–968.

Liljencrantz, J. (1922). Memory loss in the organic psychoses. *Psychol. Monogr.*, **32**, No. 143.

Lindgren, E. (1951). Encephalography in cerebral atrophy. *Acta Radiol.*, **35**, 277–291.

Lindsley, O. R. (1964). Geriatric behavioral prosthetics. In R. Kastenbaum (Ed.) *New Thoughts on Old Age*. Springer, New York.

Looft, W. R. (1973). Reflections on interaction in old age: motives, goals and assumptions. *Gerontologist*, **13**, 6–10.

Lovett-Doust, J. W., Schneider, R. A., Talland, G. A., Walsh, M. A., and Barker, G. B. (1953). Studies on the physiology of awareness: the correlation between intelligence and anoxemia in senile dementia. *J. nerv. ment. Dis.*, **117**, 383–398.

Luria, A. R. (1965). Two kinds of motor perseveration in massive injury of the frontal lobes. *Brain*, **88**, 1–10.

Luria, A. R. (1966). *Higher Cortical Functions in Man*. Tavistock, London.

McCormick, W. O. (1962). A study of the relationship between dementia and radiologically diagnosed cerebral atrophy in elderly patients. Unpublished Dissertation, University of London.

McFie, J. (1960). Psychological testing in clinical neurology. *J. nerv. ment. Dis.*, **131**, 383–393.

McGhie, A. (1973). Input dysfunction in schizophrenia. In T. J. Boag and D. Campbell (Eds) *A Triune Concept of the Brain and Behavior*. University of Toronto Press, Toronto.

McGhie, A., Chapman, J., and Lawson, J. S. (1965). Changes in immediate memory with age. *Br. J. Psychol.*, **56**, 69–75.

MacKay, H. A. (1965). Operant techniques applied to disorders of the senium. Unpublished Ph.D. Thesis, Queen's University, Kingston, Ontario.

Maddox, G., and Eisdorfer, C. (1962). Some correlates of activity and morale among the elderly. *Soc. Processes*, **40**, 228–238.

Mann, A. H. (1973). Cortical atrophy and air encephalography: a clinical and radiological study. *Psychol. Med.*, **3**, 374–378.

Marcer, D. (1974). Ageing and memory loss—role of experimental psychology. *Geront. Clin.*, **16**, 118–125.

Matarazzo, R. G., Wiens, A. N., Matarazzo, J. D., and Monaugh, T. (1973). Test–re-test reliability of the WAIS in a normal population. *J. Clin. Psychol.*, **29**, 194–197.

Matthews, C. G., and Booker, H. E. (1972). Pneumoencephalographic measurements and neuropsychological test performance in human adults. *Cortex*, **8**, 69–92.

Meehl, P. E., and Rosen, A. (1955). Antecedent probability and the efficiency of psychometric signs, patterns or cutting scores. *Psychol. Bull.*, **52**, 194–216.

Meier, M. J., and French, L. A. (1966). Longitudinal assessment of intellectual functioning following unilateral temporal lobectomy. *J. Clin. Psychol.*, **22**, 22–27.

Miller, E. (1968). A case for automated clinical testing. *Bull. Br. Psychol. Soc.*, **21**, 75–78.

Miller, E. (1971). On the nature of the memory disorder in presenile dementia. *Neuropsychologia*, **9**, 75–78.

Miller, E. (1972a). *Clinical Neuropsychology*. Penguin, Harmondsworth.

Miller, E. (1972b). Efficiency of coding and the short-term memory defect in presenile dementia. *Neuropsychologia*, **10**, 133–136.

Miller, E. (1973). Short- and long-term memory in presenile dementia (Alzheimer's disease). *Psychol. Med.*, **3**, 221–224.

Miller, E. (1974a). Psychomotor performance in presenile dementia. *Psychol. Med.*, **4**, 65–68.

Miller, E. (1974b). Retrieval from long-term memory in presenile dementia. Paper presented to Annual Conference of British Psychological Society, Bangor.

Miller, E. (1974c). Dementia as an accelerated ageing of the nervous system: some psychological and methodological considerations. *Age and Ageing*, **3**, 197–202.

Miller, E. (1975). Impaired recall and the memory disturbance in presenile dementia. *Br. J. soc. clin. Psychol.*, **14**, 73–79.

Miller, E. (1976). Visual information processing in presenile dementia. *Br. J. soc. clin. Psychol.*, in press.

Miller, E., and Hague, F. (1975). Some statistical characteristics of speech in presenile dementia. *Psychol. Med.*, **5**, 255–259.

Miner, B. (1966). Amnesia following operation on the temporal lobes. In C. W. M. Whitty and O. L. Zangwill (Eds) *Amnesia*. Butterworth, London.

Milner, B., Corkin, S., and Teuber, H.-L. (1968). Further analysis of the hippocampal amnesic syndrome: fourteen year follow-up study of HM. *Neuropsychologia*, **6**, 215–234.

Moenster, P. A. (1972). Learning and memory in relation to age. *J. Geront.*, **27**, 361–363.

Morgan, R. F. (1965). Note on the psychopathology of senility: senescent defence against the threat of death. *Psychol. Rep.*, **17**, 305–306.

Morgan, R. F. (1967). Memory and the senile psychoses: a follow-up note. *Psychol. Rep.*, **20**, 733–734.

Moore, T. V. (1919). A correlation between memory and perception in the presence of diffuse cortical degeneration. *Psychol. Monogr.*, No. 120.

Mueller, D. J., and Atlas, L. (1972). Resocialization of regressed elderly residents: a behavioral management approach. *J. Geront.*, **27**, 390–392.

Müller, H. F., and Grad, B. (1974). Clinical-psychological, electroencephalographic, and adrenocortical relationships in elderly psychiatric patients. *J. Geront.*, **27**, 237–244.

Munch-Petersen, S., Parkenberg, H., Kornerup, H., Ortmann, J., Ipsen, E., Jacobsen, P., and Simmelsgard, H. (1974). RNA treatment of dementia. *Acta Neurol. Scand.*, **50**, 553–572.

Neisser, U. (1967). *Cognitive Psychology*. Appleton-Century-Crofts, New York.

Nelson, E. H. (1953). An experimental investigation of intellectual speed and power in mental disorders. Unpublished Ph. D. Thesis, University of London.

Neugarten, B. L. (1973). Personality change in late life: a developmental perspective. In C. Eisdorfer and M. P. Lawton (Eds) *The Psychology of Adult Development and Aging*. American Psychological Association, Washington, D. C.

Neugarten, B. L., Crotty, W. F., and Tobin, S. S. (1964). *Personality in Middle and Late Life*. Atherton Press, New York.

Neugarten, B. L., Havighurst, R. J., and Tobin, S. S. (1968). Personality and patterns of aging. In B. L. Neugarten (Ed.) *Middle Age and Aging: A Reader in Social Psychology*. University of Chicago Press, Chicago.

Newcombe, F., and Steinberg, B. (1964). Some aspects of learning and memory function in older psychiatric patients. *J. Geront.*, **19**, 490–493.

Nielsen, R., Peterson, O., Thygesen, P., and Willanger, R. (1966). Encephalographic cortical atrophy. *Acta Radiol. Diagn.*, **4**, 437–448.

Norris, A. S., and Pearlman, A. (1965). Capillary morphology and performance on the trail making test in the elderly. *J. Geront.*, **20**, 76–77.

Nott, R. N., and Fleminger, J. J. (1975). Presenile dementia: the difficulties of early diagnosis. *Acta Psychiat. Scand.*, **51**, 210–217.

Noyes, A. P., and Kolb, L. C. (1958). *Modern Clinical Psychiatry.* W. B. Saunders, New York.

Oakley, D. P. (1965). Senile dementia: some aetiological factors. *Br. J. Psychiat.*, **111**, 414–419.

O'Brien, M. D., and Veall, N. (1966). Effect of cyclandelate on cerebral cortex perfusion rates in cerebrovascular disease. *Lancet*, **2**, 729–730.

Obrist, W. D., Sokoloff, L., Lassen, N. A., Lane, M. H., Buller, N. N., and Feinberg, I. (1963). Relation of EEG to cerebral blood flow and metabolism in old age. *Electroenceph. Clin. Neurophysiol.*, **15**, 610–619.

Obusek, C. J., and Warren, R. M. (1973). A comparison of speech perception in senile and well-preserved aged by means of the verbal transformation effect. *J. Geront.*, **28**, 184–188.

Olesen, J. (1974). Cerebral blood flow methods for measurement regulation: effects of drugs and changes in disease. *Acta Neurol. Scand.*, Suppl. No. 57.

O'Nell, P. M., and Calhoun, K. S. (1975). Sensory deficits and behavioral deterioration in senescence. *J. abnorm. Psychol.*, **84**, 579–582.

Orme, J. E. (1955). Intellectual and Rorschach test performances of a group of senile dementia patients and a group of elderly depressives. *J. Ment. Sci.*, **101**, 863–867.

Orme, J. E., (1957). Non-verbal and verbal performance in normal old age, senile dementia and elderly depression. *J. Geront.*, **12**, 408–413.

Owens, W. A. (1966). Age and mental abilities: a second adult follow-up. *J. Educ. Psychol.*, **57**, 311–325.

Parsons, P. L. (1965). Mental health of Swansea's old folk. *Br. J. Prev. Soc. Med.*, **19**, 43–58.

Payne, R. W. (1960). Cognitive abnormalities. In H. J. Eysenck (Ed.) *Handbook of Abnormal Psychology.* Pitman Medical, London.

Payne, R. W. (1973). Cognitive abnormalities. In H. J. Eysenck (Ed.) *Handbook of Abnormal Psychology.* 2nd ed., Pitman, London.

Payne, R. W., and Jones, H. G. (1957). Statistics for the investigation of individual cases. *J. Clin. Psychol..*, **13**, 117–121.

Pearce, J., and Miller, E. (1973). *Clinical Aspects of Dementia.* Baillière Tindall, London.

Pinkerton, P., and Kelly, J. (1952). An attempted correlation between clinical and psychometric findings in senile arteriosclerotic dementia. *J. Ment. Sci.*, **98**, 244–255.

Post, F. (1966). Somatic and psychic factors in the treatment of elderly psychiatric patients. *J. Psychosom. Res.*, **10**, 13–19.

Pressey, S. P., and Kuhlen, R. G. (1957). *Psychological Development Through the Lifespan.* Harper and Row, New York.

Quilitch, H. R. (1974). Puposeful activity increased in a geriatric ward through programmed recreation. *J. Amer. Geriat. Soc.*, **22**, 226–229.

Rabbitt, P. M. A. (1965). An age decrement in the ability to ignore irrelevant information. *J. Geront.*, **20**, 233–238.

Rabbitt, P. M. A. (1968). Age and the use of structure in transmitted information. In G. A. Talland (Ed.) *Human Aging and Behavior.* Academic Press, New York.

Rabin, A. I. (1945). Psychometric trends in senility and psychoses of the senium. *J. Gen. Psychol.*, **32**, 149–162.

Reitan, R. M. and Davison, L. A. (1974). *Clinical Neuropsychology: Current Status and Applications.* Wiley, New York.

Reynell, W. R. (1944). A psychometric method of determining intellectual loss following head injury. *J. Ment. Sci.*, **90**, 710–719.

Rochford, G. (1971). A study of naming errors in dysphasic and in demented patients. *Neuropsychologia*, **9**, 437–443.

157

Rorschach, H. (1942). *Psychodiagnostics.* Hans Huber, Berne.

Roth, M. (1955). The natural history of mental disorder in old age. *J. Ment. Sci.,* **101,** 281–301.

Roth, M., and Hopkins, B. (1953). Test performance of patients over 60. *J. Ment. Sci.,* **99,** 439–450.

Roth, M., Tomlinson, B. E., and Blessed, G. (1966). Correlation between scores for dementia and counts of senile plaques in cerebral grey matter of elderly subjects. *Nature,* **209,** 109–110.

Roth, M., Tomlinson, B. E., and Blessed, G. (1967). The relationship between quantitative measures of dementia and of degenerative changes in the cerebral grey matter of elderly subjects. *Proc. R. Soc. Med.,* **60,** 254–260.

Rothschild, D. (1937). Pathologic changes in senile psychoses and their psychobiologic significance. *Amer. J. Psychiat.,* **93,** 757–784.

Rothschild, D. (1942). Neuropathological changes in arteriosclerotic psychosis and their psychiatric significance. *Arch. Neurol. Psychiat.,* **48,** 417–436.

Rothschild, D., and Sharp, M. L. (1941). The origin of senile psychoses: neuropathologic factors and factors of a more personal nature. *Dis. Nerv. Syst.,* **2,** 49–54.

Routtenberg, A. (1968). The two-arousal hypothesis: reticular formation and limbic system. *Psychol. Rev.,* **75,** 51–80.

Sanders, H. I., and Warrington, E. K. (1971). Memory for remote events in amnesia. *Brain,* **94,** 661–668.

Sanderson, R. E. and Inglis, J. (1961). Learning and mortality in elderly psychiatric patients. *J. Geront.,* **16,** 375–376.

Savage, R. D. (1971). Psychometric assessment and clinical diagnosis in the aged. In. D. W. Kay and A. Walk (Eds) *Recent Developments in Psychogeriatrics.* Royal Medical Psychological Association, London.

Savage, R. D. (1973). Old age. In H. J. Eysenck (Ed.) *Handbook of Abnormal Psychology.* 2nd ed., Pitman, London.

Schaie, K. W., and Gribbin, K. (1975). Adult development and aging. *Ann. Rev. Psychol.,* **26,** 65–96.

Schaie, K. W., and Marquette, B. (1972). Personality in maturity and old age. In R. M. Dreger (Ed.) *Multivariate Personality Research: Contributions to the Understanding of Personality in Honour of Raymond B. Cattell.* Claitor's, Louisiana.

Schaie, K. W., and Strother, C. R. (1968a). The effect of time and cohort differences upon age changes in cognitive behavior. *Multivar. Behav. Res.,* **3,** 259–294.

Schaie, K. W., and Strother, C. R. (1968b). A cross-sequential study of age changes in cognitive behavior. *Psychol. Bull.,* **70,** 671–680.

Schonfield, D. (1967). Memory loss with age: acquisition and retrieval. *Psychol. Rep.,* **20,** 223–226.

Schonfield, D., and Robertson, B. (1966). Memory storage and aging. *Canad. J. Psychol.,* **20,** 228–236.

Shah, K. V., Banks, G. D., and Mesky, H. (1969). Survival in athersclerotic and senile dementia. *Br. J. Psychiat.,* **115,** 1283–1286.

Shakow, D., Dolkart, M. B., and Goldman, R. (1941). Memory function in psychoses of the aged. *Dis. Nerv. Syst.,* **2,** 43–48.

Shapiro, M. B., and Nelson, E. H. (1955). An investigation of the nature of cognitive impairment in co-operative psychiatric patients. *Br. J. Med. Psychol.,* **4,** 205–280.

Short, M. J., Musella, L., and Wilson, W. P. (1968). Correlation of affect and EEG in senile psychoses. *J. Geront.,* **23,** 324–327.

Simard, D., Olesen, J., Paulson, O. B., Lassen, N. A., and Skinhoj, E. (1971). Regional cerebral blood flow and its regulation in dementia. *Brain,* **94,** 273–288.

Singleton, W. T. (1954). The change in movement timing with age. *Br. J. Psychol.,* **45,** 166–172.

Sjaasted, O., and Lonnum, A. (1966). Long-term prognosis of patients with cerebral ventricular enlargement. *Acta Neurol. Scand.,* **42,** 317–353.

Sjogren, T., Sjogren, H., and Lindgren, A. G. H. (1952). Morbus Alzheimer and morbus Pick: a genetic, clinical and patho-anatomical study. *Acta Psychiat. Scand.*, Suppl. No. 82.

Slaby, A. E., and Wyatt, R. J. (1974). *Dementia in the Presenium.* C. C. Thomas, Springfield, Ill.

Slater, E., and Roth, M. (1969). *Clinical Psychiatry*. 3rd ed., Baillière Tindall, London.

Smith, A. D. (1975). Aging and interference with memory. *J. Geront.*, **30**, 319–325.

Solyom, L., and Barik, H. C. (1965). Conditioning in senescence and senility. *J. Geront.*, **20**, 483–488.

Sommer, R., and Ross, H. (1958). Social interaction on a geriatric ward. *Internat. J. Soc. Psychiat.*, **4**, 128–133.

Sperling, G. A. (1960). The information available in brief visual presentation. *Psychol. Monogr.*, **74**, No. 498.

Stengel, E. (1943). A study of the symptomatology and differential diagnosis of Alzheimer's and Pick's diseases. *J. Ment. Sci.*, **89**, 1–20.

Stengel, E. (1964). Psychopathology of dementia. *Proc. R. Soc. Med.*, **57**, 911–914.

Storck, P. A., Looft, W. R., and Hooper, F. H. (1972). Interrelationships among Piagetian tests and traditional measures of cognitive abilities in mature and aged adults. *J. Geront.*, **27**, 461–465.

Straumanis, J. J., Shagass, C., and Schwartz, M. (1965). Visually evoked response changes associated with chronic brain syndromes and ageing. *J. Geront.*, **20**, 498–506.

Taub, H. A. (1975). Mole of presentation, age, and short-term memory. *J. Geront.*, **30**, 56–59.

Taulbee, L. R., and Folsom, J. C. (1966). Reality orientation for geriatric patients. *Hosp. Commun. Psychiat.*, **17**, 133–135.

Thaler, M. (1956). Relationships among Wechsler, Weigl, Rorschach, EEG findings and abstract–concrete behavior in a group of normal aged subjects. *J. Geront.*, **11**, 404–409.

Thorndike, E. L., and Lorge, I. (1944). *The Teacher's Word Book of 30,000 Words*. Teacher's College, Columbia University, New York.

Thurstone, L. L. (1938). Primary mental abilities. *Psychol. Monogr.*, **51**, No. 3.

Thurstone, L. L., and Thurstone, T. G. (1946). *S. R. A. Primary Mental Abilities. Ages 11 to 17*. Science Research Associates, Chicago.

Tomlinson, B. E., Blessed, G., and Roth, M. (1970). Observations on the brains of demented old people. *J. Neurol. Sci.*, **7**, 205–242.

Turland, D. N., and Steinhard, M. (1969). The efficiency of the Memory-for-Designs test. *Br. J. soc. clin. Psychol.*, **8**, 44–49.

Uecker, A. E. (1969). Comparability of two methods of administering the MMPI to brain damaged geriatric patients. *J. Clin. Psychol.*, **25**, 196–198.

Walton, D., and Black, D. A. (1957). The validity of a psychological test of brain damage. *Br. J. med. Psychol.*, **20**, 270–279.

Walton, D., White, J. G., Black, D. A., and Young, A. J. (1959). The modified word learning test—a cross validation study. *Br. J. Med. Psychol.*, **22**, 213–220.

Wang, H. S., Obrist, W. D., and Busse, E. W. (1970). Neurophysiological correlates of the intellectual function of elderly persons living in the community. *Amer. J. Psychiat.*, **126**, 1205–1215.

Wang, H. S., and Whanger, A. (1971). Brain impairment and longevity. In E. Palmore and F. C. Jeffers (Eds) *Prediction of Life Span*, Heath Lexington Books, Lexington, Mass.

Warren, R. M., and Gregory, R. L. (1958). An auditory analogue of the visual reversible figure. *Amer. J. Psychol.*, **71**, 612–613.

Warrington, E. K. (1970). Neurological deficits. In P. J. Mittler (Ed.) *The Psychological Assessment of Mental and Physical Handicap*. Methuen, London.

Warrington, E. K., and Weiskrantz, L. (1970). Amneisc syndrome: consolidation or retrieval? *Nature*, **228**, 628–630.

Warrington, E. K., and Weiskrantz, L. (1971). Organizational aspects of memory in amnesic patients. *Neuropsychologia*, **9**, 67–73.

Waugh, N. C., Fozard, J. L., Talland, G. A., and Erwin, D. E. (1973). Effects of age and stimulus repetition on two-choice reaction time. *J. Geront.*, **28**, 466–470.

Wechsler, D. (1945). A standardised memory scale for clinical use, *J. Psychol.*, **19**, 87–95.

Wechsler, D. (1955). *Manual for the Wechsler Adult Intelligence Scale.* The Psychological Corporation, New York.

Wechsler, D. (1958). *The Measurement and Appraisal of Adult Intelligence.* Williams and Wilkins, Baltimore.

Welford, A. T. (1959). Psychomotor performance. In J. E. Birren (Ed.) *Handbook of Aging and the Individual.* University of Chicago Press, Chicago.

Welford, A. T. (1962). On changes of movement timing with age. *Lancet*, **1**, 335–339.

Wetherick, N. E. (1966). The inferential basis of concept attainment. *Br. J. Psychol.*, **57**, 61–69.

Whanger, A. D., and Wang, H. S. (1974). Clinical correlates of the vibratory sense in elderly psychiatric patients. *J. Geront.*, **29**, 39–45.

White, A. R. (1967). *The Philosophy of Mind.* Random House, New York.

White, J. G., Merrick, M., and Harbison, J. J. M. (1969). William's scale for the measurement of memory: test reliability and validity in a psychiatric population. *Br. J. soc. clin. Psychol.*, **8**, 141–151.

Whitehead, A. (1973a). Verbal learning and memory in elderly depressives. *Br. J. Psychiat.*, **123**, 203–208.

Whitehead, A. (1973b). The pattern of WAIS performance in elderly psychiatric patients. *Br. J. soc. clin. Psychol.*, **12**, 435–436.

Whitehead, A. (1975). Recognition memory in dementia. *Br. J. soc. clin. Psychol.*, **14**, 191–194.

Wickelgren, W. A. (1968). Sparing of short-term memory in the amnesic patient: Implications for strength theory of memory. *Neuropsychologia*, **6**, 235–244.

Wilkie, F., and Eisdorfer, C. (1971). Intelligence and blood pressure in the aged. *Science*, **172**, 959–962.

Willanger, R. (1970a). The relation between anamnestic information about intellectual functions and cerebral atrophy. *Acta Neurol. Scand.*, Suppl. No. 43.

Willanger, R. (1970b). *Intellectual Impairment in Diffuse Cerebral Lesions.* Munksgaard, Copenhagen.

Willanger, R., and Klee, A. (1966). Metamorphosia and other visual disturbances with latency occurring in patients with diffuse cerebral lesions. *Acta Neurol. Scand.*, Suppl. No. 42.

Willanger, R., Thygesen, P., Nielsen, R., and Petersen, O. (1968). Intellectual impairment and cerebral atrophy: a psychological, neurological and radiological investigation. *Dan. Med. Bull.*, **15**, 65–93.

Williams, H. W., Quesnel, E., Fish, V. W., and Goodman, L. (1942). Studies in senile and arteriosclerotic psychoses. 1. Relative significance of extrinsic factors in their development. *Amer. J. Psychiat.*, **98**, 712–715.

Williams, M. (1956a). Studies of perception in senile dementia: cue selection as a function of intelligence. *Br. J. Med. Psychol.*, **19**, 270–279.

Williams, M. (1956b). Spatial disorientation in senile dementia. *J. Ment. Sci.*, **102**, 291–299.

Williams, M. (1965). *Mental Testing in Clinical Practice.* Pergamon Press, New York.

Williams, M. (1968). The measurement of memory in clinical practice. *Br. J. soc. clin. Psychol.*, **7**, 19–34.

Wilson, D. C. (1955). The pathology of senility. *Amer. J. Psychiat.*, **111**, 902–906.

Wolfensberger, W. (1970). The principle of normalization and its implications for psychiatric services. *Amer. J. Psychiat.*, **127**, 291–297.

Wolfensberger, W. (1972). *The Principle of Normalization in Human Services.* National Institute on Mental Retardation, Toronto.

Wood, J. H., Bartlett, D., James, A. E., and Udvarhelyi, G. B. (1974). Normal pressure hydrocephalus: diagnosis and patient selection for surgery. *Neurology*, **24**, 517–526.

160

Yacorzynski, G. K. (1941). An evaluation of the postulates underlying the Babcock deterioration test. *Psychol. Rev.*, **48**, 261–267.

Yates, A. J. (1954). The validity of some psychological tests of brain damage. *Psychol. Bull.*, **51**, 359–379.

Yates, A. J. (1956). The use of vocabulary in the measurement of intellectual deterioration—a review. *J. Ment. Sci.*, **102**, 409–440.

Young, J., Hall, P., and Blakemore, C. B. (1974). Treatment of the cerebral manifestations of arteriosclerosis with cyclandelate. *Br. J. Psychiat.*, **124**, 177–180.

Zangwill, O. L. (1964). Psychopathology of dementia. *Proc. R. Soc. Med.*, **57**, 914–917.

Zipf, G. K. (1949). *Human Behaviour and the Principle of Least Effort*. Addison Wesley, New York.

Author Index

Subject Index